CMA Study Guide 2020-2021

CMA Exam Preparation with 600 Questions and Detailed Answer Explanations for the Certified Medical Assistant Exam (6 Full Practice Tests)

Table of Contents

Background Information

A medical assistant is otherwise known as a health-care assistant or clinical assistant. This is a health professional who is responsible for working with physicians and other medical professionals as an assistant.

Medical assistants perform some routine procedures and tasks that make the work of health professionals a lot easier. You can find medical assistants in hospitals, working with physicians, or in other health-care facilities where they perform clinical and administrative tasks.

Medical assistants perform the following tasks:

- Measure blood pressure and other vital signs
- Record patients' personal information and history
- Perform patient examinations for physicians
- Update medical records with patients' information
- Book-keeping
- Assist physicians with diagnostic examinations
- Prepare patients for tests and examinations
- File and update patients' medical records
- Handle correspondence
- Answer telephone calls
- File insurance forms
- Schedule appointments
- Stock exam rooms
- Perform vision screening, EKGs and other specialized tests
- Collect specimens for lab tests

<u>Documenting and Managing Medical Records.</u>

Note that your job description as a medical assistant is dependent on the laws of the jurisdiction of your employment.

Irrespective of your state of employment, you will work directly under the supervision of a licensed nurse or doctor.

Medical assistants are needed in:

- Outpatient care centers
- Offices of medical health practitioners
- Hospitals

- Offices of chiropractors

Certification affords medical assistants opportunities that are not available to non-certified medical assistants.

Sometimes medical assistants are mistaken for physician assistants. However, these are two distinct professions.

While a physician assistant is trained and licensed to perform surgical operations and practice medicine together with a trained physician, medical assistants only perform routine procedures and tasks.

Qualities of a Medical Assistant

Medical assistants are expected to possess some qualities that are crucial to their success in their chosen profession. As a medical assistant, you must have:

Interpersonal Skills: Your interpersonal skills must be excellent as a medical assistant. You must be able to have clear discussions about patients with physicians. This is aside from your ability to interact meaningfully and comfortingly with distressed patients.

Analytical Skills: While assisting physicians, you are required to understand diagnoses and medical charts.

Technical Skills: Your job isn't limited to updating records. Rather, it also involves taking a patient's vital signs such as blood pressure, heart rate and more.

Verbal Communication: Checking vital signs, conveying messages to patients and generally working with medical personnel places a huge responsibility on you. Your verbal communication skills must be outstanding to enable you to discharge your responsibilities satisfactorily.

Organizational Skills: Maintaining organized medical records is crucial to the success of a medical procedure. Doctors always refer to such records during treatments. Thus, you should be able to retrieve a record whenever it is needed.

Infection Control Skills: Coming into contact with bodily fluids and blood makes you susceptible to infection. You may infect other patients as well if you don't take infection control seriously.

A section of this book is dedicated to infection control. The section provides some practical tips that can assist you in staying safe while discharging your responsibilities.

Developing these six skill sets will make you invaluable to the physicians you assist, and that will have a huge positive impact on your career.

Education and Licensing Requirements

To become a medical assistant, you must possess the required level of education, have the right working experience and meet some licensing requirements.

This is a short list of the basic requirements:

- You must be a certified clinical medical assistant (CCMA
- You must possess a minimum of one year's work experience as a medical assistant
- You must be familiar with medical terminology
- You must be experienced at using electronic medical records (EMR)

However, you have a better chance of climbing the career ladder faster if you get the necessary certification. This is because certification is a requirement by many recruiters and organizations.

This highlights the importance of the Certified Medical Assistance certification administered by the American Association of Medical Assistants (AAMA).

The objective of this book is to prepare you for the CMA examination. The next section of the book provides some invaluable information that will help you prepare for the exam as well as provide some practical tips that will boost your chances of success.

General Section

This section reviews the CMA exam rules, format, dos and don'ts and other key information pertaining to the exam.

Test Format

The CMA exam is computerized. Students can choose to take the test at any number of Prometric centers around the world.

The examination consists of 180 scored and 20 unscored multiple-choice questions. Each question has four answers to choose from.

Time to Take the Test

Each student has 160 minutes to attempt the 200 questions. The exam is divided into four segments, each assigned 40 minutes.

Since the test is computer-based, the computer automatically logs you out of a session once the allotted time is up, regardless of whether you have completed the session or not. Thus, speed and accuracy are vital while taking the exam.

The questions are drawn from the following categories:

- Administrative section: 45 questions
- General section: 50 questions
- Clinical section: 85 questions

Now that you are aware of the time limits, you can better prepare for the exam.

Eligibility for the Examination

The CMA examination is not open to the general public. Furthermore, it is not available to everyone in the medical profession.

To be eligible, you must fall into any of these three classes:

Category 1: In this category are students who recently graduated from any accredited medical assisting program.

Individuals may take the CMA certification examination at least 30 days after graduating from the program. The examination must be completed within a year of graduation.

Program completion must be verified by the program director.

Category 2: In this category are candidates who graduated from an accredited medical assistant program more than a year ago. Such candidates are required to submit their official transcript in order to determine whether they are qualified to test.

Category 3: The final category involves candidates who have previously passed the CMA exam and wish to be recertified. They are expected to provide their CMA certificate numbers or any recent recertification or certification date.

In a nutshell, your eligibility for the examination is dependent on passing medical assistant programs accredited by the Accrediting Bureau of Health Education Schools or the Commission on Accreditation of Allied Health Education Programs.

How to Register for the Exam

Once you meet the basic eligibility requirements, you can proceed to the AAMA's website to submit your application form.

You will be charged a $125 application fee. Note that this fee is neither transferable nor refundable and depends on the eligibility category you fall in.

These are the candidate fees according to categories:

- Category 1 – $125
- Categories 2 and 3 – $125 or $250 for AAMA members and non-members respectively.

You can pay by debit or credit card. A certified cashier's check, money order or institution check is also accepted for payment. Personal checks are not accepted.

After payment, the certification department will email you an update on your status within 30 days.

Once your application request is approved, log into the AAMA's website to print your scheduling permit. You need the permit to schedule your test.

You can forfeit the assigned 90-day testing period for the scheduling permit if you don't complete your registration. An "incomplete" status on your registration page is a reminder of what you must do to complete the registration.

If you miss the testing period, you must reapply for the examination. You will have to pay the exam fee again.

Where to Take the Test

You can choose any of the approved Prometric centers for the examination. Since there are many options to choose from, it is advisable that you choose a center within your neighborhood.

Test times and dates are usually on a first-come, first-served basis. Therefore, apply for the examination as soon as possible to ensure you can test on your preferred date and at the most convenient location.

What to Do on Test Day

For starters, arrive at the center at least 30 minutes before the examination time. Tardiness will automatically disqualify you from taking the test.

Bring a valid identification card to the testing center. Ensure that every piece of information on your ID tallies matches the information you supplied during registration. Irregularities in the information will disqualify you from testing. For example, your name on your ID should match your name on the application.

Don't take anything like cell phones, notes or other personal belongings into the test center. They are not allowed, and if you are caught with them, you will be disqualified from taking the test.

What Students Can Do

As a student, you can do a lot of things that make it easier for you to pass the examination.

- Arrive at the test center early
- Prepare thoroughly for the exam
- Apply early for the exam

What Students Cannot Do

Do not:

- Arrive late at the exam center
- Bring personal items into the center
- Leave the testing room without permission

Passing Score

The passing score is 430.

At the end of the test, the examination body will give you an official fail/pass notification. This is just to provide you with a general overview of your performance on the exam. However, you will receive an official performance result within a week of taking the test.

The report will include a breakdown of your performance in percentiles. Three categories of the test will be considered for the ranking: Administrative, General and Clinical. The information will enable you to identify your weaknesses and strengths. Thus, you will know quickly whether you need to retake the exam or not.

If you pass the exam, you will receive the CMA (AAMA) credential as proof of your certification.

Cancel/Reschedule

Each candidate for the examination is given 90 days to schedule and take the exam. The 90-day period depends on when you apply for the exam. Candidates who apply for it during the first 14 days of the month will start their grace period on the first day of the next month. Applicants from the 15th of the month to the end of the month will start their 90-day period on the 15th of the next month.

After your application, the body will give you a scheduling permit. Visit the AAMA's website to schedule your exam. Alternatively, you can schedule the exam by calling the number on your permit.

If you can't take the examination within the 90-day period, you automatically forfeit your registration fee and will need to pay a $65 penalty to schedule during the next period.

If you do not pass the exam, you can retake it after 90 days. You will have to repeat the registration process and pay the necessary fees again.

Each candidate has a maximum of three opportunities to attempt the exam. Failure to pass on the third try means you will never be able to become a certified CMA.

Tips to Help You Pass the CMA Exam

You can boost your chances to pass the exam by:

- Carefully studying this book
- Reviewing the Questions and Answers sections thoroughly
- Identifying weaknesses and working to strengthen them
- Setting aside some time every day to study

Chapter One: Medical Law/Regulatory Guidelines

Some of the most important regulatory guidelines and medical laws you will need to know as a medical assistant are:

Advance Directives

An advance directive informs medical practitioners of the type of treatment a patient accepts or doesn't accept. The directive is always valid even if the patient is unconscious or lacks the physical or mental strength to make his or her wishes known.

The most common advance directives are:

The Living Will

This is a legal document that reflects a person's future health-care decisions in the event that the person can't make valid choices or decisions due to poor health or any other factors.

It is the reference point for health decisions for terminally ill people or people who are permanently unconscious and thus don't have the physical or mental ability to make health-care decisions.

In a living will, the person's preferred medical treatment is documented. The living will also lists the type of medical treatment the individual rejects. It lists the conditions that warrant that the sick person's life should be prolonged through medical means or when treatment should be discontinued.

Some major medical information contained in the living will is related to tube feeding, dialysis and life support.

Before the living will is made, two physicians must have appraised the patient's health and ascertained that he/she can't make his/her own medical decisions. That is particularly applicable if the patient's condition falls under the category specified by state law as either permanent unconsciousness or terminal illness.

The living will may be considered when making some important health decisions such as:

- Whether to use dialysis machine or ventilators
- Treatment for health conditions even if a patient can't personally make such decisions
- Whether to use IV or tube feeding if drinking or eating is difficult or impossible
- Organ and/or tissue donation after death

- Whether or not CPR should be administered

Durable Power of Attorney

The durable power of attorney is otherwise known as medical power of attorney. It is a legal document that a patient uses to transfer major health-care decisions to a proxy or an agent if the patient becomes incapacitated and is unable to make such decisions.

This legal document becomes the major medium for making health-related decisions when a patient's decision has certified that the person in question lacks the ability to make medical decisions for him or herself. Some of the aforementioned health problems may be responsible for such a transfer of decision-making to a third party.

The proxy and the patient must be familiar with each other to enable them to make accurate health decisions on behalf of the sick individual. They should understand how the patient would likely make decisions if he/she had the capability to do so.

Hence, people are always advised to discuss their health concerns and decisions with such agents while they are able to do so.

Note that laws governing durable power of attorney differ from one state to another. Thus, a patient is advised to be familiar with the laws of his/her state when drafting a power of attorney.

Patient Self-Determination Act

In 1990, the United States Congress passed the Patient Self-Determination Act (PSDA) as a replacement for a previous act, the Omnibus Budget Reconciliation Act of 1990. The legislation made it mandatory for health agencies such as nursing homes, hospitals, home health agencies and other health-care provides to provide adult patients with sufficient information about existing advance health-care directives.

Once an adult is admitted to a health-care facility, the patient should be provided with a written notice that spells out the facility's policies and the individual's decision-making rights within the confines of the state's law.

The notice should detail patients':

- Right to refuse or accept any form of medical treatment
- Right to make health-care decisions for themselves
- Right to opt for advance health-care directives

The facility must ask patients whether they have advanced health-care directives or not. The response must be fully documented for future reference.

Health-care facilities must also educate staff about existing advance health-care directives.

The primary objective of the Patient Self-Determination Act is to ensure that patients are not kept in the dark about their health. Patients should be fully informed about their rights to make personal decisions that affect their health through the type of medical treatment they accept or reject.

Some health conditions that may deprive someone of the power to make medical decisions include:

- Being in a coma
- Being in a persistent vegetative state
- Cognitive damage caused by a stroke
- Loss of communication ability
- Moderate or severe Alzheimer's or any other form of dementia
- Kidney failure or any other severe medical condition

Health Insurance Portability and Accountability Act

The Health Insurance Portability and Accountability Act (HIPAA) was enacted in 1996 by the US Congress to amend previous laws such as the Public Health Service Act (PHSA) and the Employee Retirement Income Security Act (ERISA).

The act set the industry standard for how patients' information is used and shared in an effort to ensure the protection of patients' personal medical data. The act helps prevent identify theft and/or fraud by keeping medical information private.

HIPAA impacts technology, policies and record-keeping acts at health insurance companies, medical facilities, health-care billing services and HMOs.

Noncompliance with this act is considered a criminal offense.

HIPAA Uses and Disclosure

Certain types of patient information may be disclosed if absolutely necessary for these situations and purposes:

- For payment, treatment and health-care procedures
- For public interest. Under the HIPAA Privacy Rule, health-care providers are permitted to disclose protected health information when required by the law, to prevent a threat to a patient's safety or as needed by some government functions.

Patient Care Partnership/Patient's Bill of Rights

Sometimes, patients don't know the expectations of their medical team. It is also not uncommon for patients to have high expectations of their physicians. Either of the two situations may cause friction between patients and health-care providers.

In 2003, the American Hospital Association enacted the Patient Care Partnership to address this situation and help patients to have a balanced view of their expectations and thus establish a good physician/patient relationship. The Patient Care Partnership also addresses patient rights and responsibilities when receiving treatment in a health-care facility.

The document highlights the importance of good communication between the medical team and a patient. Patients are free to express their opinions and reservations. They must be provided with answers to their questions so they can accept or reject treatment.

The document highlights some key health-care facility responsibilities:

- A clean environment: Cleanliness is a requirement for all health facilities.
- A safe environment: Under no circumstance should a patient ever feel his/her safety is threatened when receiving medical attention in any facility.
- Optimum protection of privacy: Both federal and state laws require health- care facilities to protect their patients' privacy. Hence, they don't have the liberty to use personal information for their personal benefit and cannot share such information with a third party unless it is absolutely necessary.
- High-quality hospital care: Patients deserve nothing but the best medical attention. This is made clear in the document.
- Patients should be involved in their own care: Patients must be involved when decisions about their health are discussed. Thus, they have the right to turn down health procedures they are not comfortable with.

Hence, health-care providers should discuss treatment plans with patients as well as relevant medical decisions. The discussion should include the risks and benefits of each treatment option available. The potential long-term effects of the treatment must be part of this discussion.

A patient's responsibilities include:

- Providing health-care services with personal information that may assist with treatment. The information should include pain, current symptoms and medications, if any
- Asking relevant questions that may help the patient be better able to make informed decisions

- Inform health-care providers of any appointment cancelations as early as possible

Consent to Treatment

Patients must give express permission before they are given any type of medical test, treatment or examination.

The physician should keep the patient in the loop before consent is sought. Thus, the patient must know the reason for a specific treatment or procedure. It is immaterial whether the patient is considering organ donation or physical examination; consent must still be sought before any treatment is administered.

The principle has become crucial to the medical community and is considered important in terms of human rights law.

Consent can only be considered valid if it meets two conditions. It must be informed and voluntary. Thus, the decision to consent to treatment or not must not be forced. The person must personally make the decision without undue interference or pressure by friends, medical staff or family.

Consent must also be an informed decision. All information involving the treatment must be specifically spelled out. Are there alternatives? What about the risks and benefits of the treatment? What are the likely consequences of not going ahead with the treatment? All this information, and any other applicable details, must be fully explained to the patient.

Does the person have the mental capacity to make the decision and give consent?

Patients are considered to have the capacity to make important health-care decisions if they meet the following conditions:

- They understand the information that is relevant to the health decision they are about to make
- They have the ability to retain whatever information they are provided with
- They can effectively use any communication means to make their decisions known
- They have the ability to weigh the information before making a decision

If a patient doesn't meet any of the four criteria outlined above, he/she is deemed unfit to give consent (or to deny it).

However, if someone can't make a decision due to deteriorating health, the power of attorney may be invoked. Alternatively, if there are no provisions for a power of attorney, the physician can proceed with the treatment if there are no doubts that the treatment will serve the patient's interest.

A patient can give either verbal or written consent. In the former, the patient may verbally indicate a willingness to accept the treatment, while the latter involves signing a consent form. A typical example is surgery. Most patients sign a consent form before a surgical operation is performed on them.

However, there are some exceptions to the rule. The health-care provider may not need any form of consent under these conditions:

- If there is an emergency that requires urgent treatment to save the person's life and he/she is incapacitated and can't give consent at the time
- If the patient has a serious mental problem such as bipolar disorder, schizophrenia, dementia and other related health problems
- If the patient is a cholera or rabies patient. People with tuberculosis also fall into this class. Since such individuals may constitute a huge risk to public health, it is not mandatory that they give written or verbal consent before they are treated
- If the sick person is living in an environment that may worsen his/her health condition. An example is someone living in unsanitary conditions where treatment is almost impossible. The patient's consent isn't needed to take him/her to a better location.

While consent giving is the patient's responsibility, when it comes to minors, parents may make decisions on their behalf without seeking their consent if such decisions are for the minors' good.

Types of Consent

There are different types of consent. These are:

Verbal Consent: Involves the patient verbally agreeing for the medical team to proceed with a treatment provided that such a treatment doesn't pose any significant risk that may further impair the patient's health.

Implied Consent: Involves cooperating with the physician's instructions, especially abiding by some routine procedures. Examples of implied consent abound. They include blood pressure tests, blood-sample taking and using medications.

Written Consent: Implies appending a signature to a document as proof of a patient's willingness to allow the physician to proceed with any procedure or treatment that may either carry a high risk or is very complex. A surgical procedure is such a treatment.

These guidelines guide the medical profession, and compliance with them is crucial to a medical professional's success.

Chapter Two: Medical Ethics

The medical profession, like every other profession, is guided and regulated by some ethics. Medical ethics consists of a set of values that serve as a reference point for medical professionals.

Principles of Medical Ethics

Medical ethics hinges on four major principles. These are:

Principle of Respect for Autonomy

Respect for autonomy implies that patients should be given the freedom to make decisions that will impact their health.

Such decisions shouldn't be made in the dark. Rather, patients must have a full understanding of the situation in order to enable them to make an informed decision.

Furthermore, patients should be allowed to voluntarily make decisions without external influences that may force them into making decisions they otherwise wouldn't have made. This principle is behind the concept of informed consent previously discussed.

Principle of Nonmaleficence

Nonmaleficence stipulates that health-care providers should be cautious of their actions. Under no condition must such actions intentionally pose a threat to their patients, whether deliberately or accidentally.

To ensure this, medical practitioners are advised to stick to the best professional standards to minimize patients' exposure to risks.

While the principle recognizes medical mistakes are inevitable, the goal is to ensure that such mistakes don't pose a big threat to patients' health or life. Their safety and security must be prioritized.

In some situations, pain may be inevitable. A typical example is a painful medical process that may prolong the patient's life. While pain may not be completely avoided, the overall objective is to make the patient healthier and not compromise his/her health or complicate issues.

Within the principle of nonmaleficence is the principle of double effect. The principle is born out of the fact that a single action may have both a bad effect and a good effect simultaneously. Thus, the principle stipulates that if an action that is morally wrong also has a morally bad consequence, it is still considered ethically okay to perform the action, provided the bad side won't override the good side and the bad side effect isn't intended. In most cases, the bad side effect is known prior to performing the action.

Some factors must be considered when considering the principle of double effect. The governing factors that deserve attention are:

- The intended good result must be achieved without depending on the bad side effect. Thus, the good effect must be independent of the bad effect and the bad effect shouldn't be the only means of achieving the good effect. The principle is invalid if a drug will kill a patient in order to perform its desired result.
- The cause and action must be proportional to each other. Medical practitioners must provide proportional medical treatment for a patient's ailment. Such treatment should be certain to give only the desired result. Hence, giving a patient an overdose of a drug violates this principle.
- Medical care must be appropriate: Aside from giving patients treatments that are proportional to their ailments, medical care must also be appropriate. You can't treat malaria with pregnancy drugs, for example.

Four conditions usually apply to the principle. These are:

- The action mustn't be morally wrong itself
- The bad effect mustn't determine the good effect
- The intention of the agent must be purely benevolent
- The good effect of the action must outweigh its bad side effect

The Principle of Beneficence

This principle stipulates that health-care providers should engage in actions that are beneficial to their patients. Thus, they must do everything possible to ensure the patient's safety and security and should go as far as to remove potential harm.

Don't mistake this with nonmaleficence. Although the principles are seemingly similar, nonmaleficence forbids health-care practitioners from harming their patients, while beneficence involves removing potential harm.

Principle of Justice

In the medical field, justice denotes a form of fairness. This implies that health-care experts should act in fairness to their patients. This principle has some connection to equality and entitlement.

In the health-care profession, the principle of justice is subdivided into three parts. These are:

- Respect for people's rights
- Fair distribution of scarce resources
- Respect for acceptable laws

Unfortunately, equal treatment isn't always administered in real-life situations. This is due to a wide range of factors that may determine how a medical practitioner responds to issues.

Some common determinants include social status, age, ethnic background, place of residence, sexual preferences, culture, legal capacity, insurance coverage and a host of other related factors. It is not uncommon for wealthy people to get the best available medical treatment, while individuals of fewer financial means may not have access to such high-quality treatment.

People are also not treated with equality when receiving medical assistance. While some are treated with respect, others are subjected to unfriendly treatment. They have to cope with indifference and rudeness from time to time.

Prejudice, racism, poverty and sexism are some of the major factors that influence some medical practitioners' attitudes toward their patients.

Medical Codes of Conduct

Some notable codes that have regulated medical ethics for decades include:

The Hippocratic Oath

This centuries-old Greek medical text ranks among the most widely known oaths that guide the medical field. Originally, it required new medical practitioners to uphold the profession and provide assurance of their determination to do so by swearing by some healing gods.

Over the years, the oath has become responsible for the establishment of several principles that guide medical ethics, including the principles of nonmaleficence and medical confidentiality.

While the former has been discussed previously, the latter establishes a rule of confidentiality that regulates the conversations between patients and doctors. During such discussions, physicians are under oath to refrain from revealing confidential information their patients share with them, even if the law requires them to share such information.

In many parts of the world, the Hippocratic oath is considered sacrosanct, a non-negotiable part of the medical profession.

The Declaration of Helsinki

The World Medical Association (WMA) specifically developed the Declaration of Helsinki (DoH) in 1964 to regulate the activities of the medical community. It contains some ethical principles that guide human experimentation for medical practitioners.

It should be noted that all physicians are under the declaration. It is morally binding on everyone in the medical field. Its importance lies in its superiority over local or national regulations or laws.

The Nuremberg Code

The Nuremberg Code was created in 1947 after the Nuremberg Trials that followed World War II.

The first of these trials, known as the Doctors' Trial, was conducted in 1947 under the Nuremberg Military Tribunals. At the trial, 23 physicians were tried for a wide range of crimes against humanity they committed during the war. These physicians turned Jewish prisoners into guinea pigs for various experiments, regardless of the prisoners' resistance to such experiments.

Sixteen of the 23 doctors were found guilty of the crimes, and seven of them were given the death penalty. Nine other doctors received various jail terms, ranging from 10 years behind bars to life imprisonment. Only seven of the doctors were acquitted.

The verdict gave physicians a reason for creating the Nuremberg Code. The 10-code ethical principle is designed to control human experimentation.

The 10 codes include:

- Voluntary consent is a requirement for any medical experimentation
- An experiment must be conducted for the general benefit of society
- Animal experimentation should form the basis for human experiments
- Experiments should be conducted in a manner and an environment that prevents mental or physical injury or suffering to humans
- Experiments with high potential for causing disability or death should be terminated
- The risks of an experiment shouldn't outweigh its benefits
- The experiment should be conducted in appropriate facilities
- The subjects of the experiment should have the choice of terminating their participation at their convenience
- Only qualified scientists should conduct the experiments
- If there is the potential for disability, injury or death, the scientist in charge of the experiment should terminate it without delay

Factors Affecting Ethical Decisions

Ethical decision-making can be affected by moral and legal factors.

Legal Factors: Legal factors are defined by local or international laws guiding the medical profession. They play a role in determining what is acceptable and what is not to medical practitioners.

Moral Factors: Moral factors are defined by values and cultural norms. Most employees pick some moral values from their immediate culture, environment, religion or education. These factors determine what is considered good or bad.

The idea of what constitutes bad or good behavior also reflects on people's general attitude, including their decision-making.

Environmental Safety

Aside from medical staff, other employees, patients and their visitors, the medical environment also must also be devoid of any danger to workers and patients. This includes:

Electrical Safety

Modern medical facilities are run on electrical devices. For instance, automated blood pressure cuffs, electric beds, diagnostic instruments and scanning equipment are some of the equipment that is powered by electricity.

This increases patients' risk of electric shock. The addition of electrode gel and some conductive solutions when patients are connected to EKG pads, defibrillation pads, patient monitors and ultrasound equipment also reduces the patients' resistance to such shocks.

This highlights why medical facilities should have effective measures in place to reduce their patients' vulnerability to electrical shock triggered by their devices. It is advisable that hospitals test their devices on grounded power systems with a view to identifying their shock risks and correcting the problem before it is too late.

The National Fire Protection Association (NFPA) has created a standard for all health-care facilities to comply with. It requires that devices used for patient care undergo leakage tests on a grounded alternating current power system in order to reduce the risks of electric shock.

In the same vein, OSHA Standard 1910 also establishes a list of grounding requirements and work practices that should be enforced in medical facilities to ensure patients and employees are safe from electrical shock.

Ergonomics

When the capacity of a worker is compared with the physical requirement of the individual's job, some health issues such as work-related musculoskeletal disorders can be prevented.

Hospital employees are not immune to job-related health problems. They are most often exposed to ligament tears, muscle strain, tendon inflammation, herniated discs, pinched nerves and other ergonomic problems that may arise as a result of transferring or handling patients frequently.

OSHA recommends that medical care providers should only lift patients when absolutely necessary. They should also minimize the number of patients they lift manually if eliminating lifting completely isn't possible.

To achieve this, medical facilities can equip their employees with wheelchairs, gait belts, sliding boards, shower chairs and other devices that reduce unnecessary musculoskeletal stress.

Medical facilities should also ensure that sufficient staff are on hand to perform a task that may be too difficult for one person, such as repositioning or transferring a patient.

Fire Prevention Regulations

Fire outbreaks can destroy a medical facility completely and put people's lives at risk. Thus, fire prevention is an integral part of all medical staff's job description.

Note that fire can't start in the absence of these three things:

A source of ignition or heat: A source of heat. This includes lighting, heaters, naked flames, matches, electrical equipment, cigarettes, etc.

A source of fuel: Fire may be fueled by paper, wood, rubber, trash, plastic and furniture.

Oxygen: Fire requires oxygen.

Fire Prevention Tips

You can prevent a fire outbreak if you implement the following fire prevention tips:

- Reduce the amount of explosive or flammable substances in the medical facility

- Keep sources of fuel or heat where people can't get easy access to them
- Prohibit smoking within medical facilities
- Ensure that sprinkler systems and alarms are available and functional

If these tips are implemented, you will minimize fire outbreaks to the barest minimum.

Chapter Three: Risk Management

The medical profession, like every other profession, has its share of risks. Thus, risk management is one of the most important skills every health-care provider must have.

Let's take a look at some practical ways health-care professionals can prevent accidents in the workplace.

Safety Symbols and Signs

The workplace, especially a medical facility, should be the place where patients not only find a solution to their health challenges but also have their safety is guaranteed.

The nature of the job increases medical workers' exposure to hazardous substances. This calls for measures that guarantee the safety of health-care providers. Thus, it is imperative that some safety precautions are put in place to ensure health workers' safety as well as the safety of patients and visitors.

Some important safety precautions in medical facilities are discussed below.

Radiation Hazards

Hospitals use some devices that utilize powerful radiation to treat a wide range of ailments. Ultrasounds, X-rays and CT scans are some of these devices. Excessive exposure to radiation is unhealthy and can trigger health issues such as cancer.

Hence, the public, medical teams and other hospital staff should all be notified of the possibility of exposure to harmful radiation. Such information will enable them to take necessary safety precautions that will reduce their exposure.

Slip and Cleaning Hazard Signs

In medical environments, hygiene is taken seriously, with good reason. Nevertheless, it is equally important that health workers and others are not exposed to unnecessary cleaning hazards by putting in place signs that warn of possible danger during cleaning. For instance, a sign may warn people of the danger of a wet floor they might otherwise slip on.

Visual instructions should be put in strategic places where they can easily be seen. This will ensure that patients, staff and visitors are not unconsciously putting themselves in danger.

Laboratory and Biohazard Signs

People's vulnerability to infectious diseases and biological hazards is heightened around medical facilities. Thus, people are more prone to coming into contact with infectious materials. Therefore, it is vital to have some relevant safety signs in place to notify health workers, patients and their visitors of the need to steer clear of such materials. This prevents infectious diseases from spreading in the facility.

Fire and Emergency Signs

One of the greatest risks that hospitals and other medical facilities have to contend with is fire. Aside from the havoc it can wreak, fire can also trigger confusion and panic, two other factors that may lead to injuries and death.

With the help of conspicuous emergency and fire signs, such as clearly marked fire exits, people within a medical facility can easily escape during an emergency.

Workplace Accident Prevention

Medical personnel may be involved in workplace accidents such as slips or falls that may undermine their health. In some instances, workplace falls result in serious health problems such as broken limbs, fractured arms and occasionally, death.

Nonfatal incidents and workplace infections are common among health-care staff too. They regularly have to contend with laser dangers, latex risks, back pain, radioactive materials, blood-borne pathogens and work environment stress, among others.

Workplace accidents can be prevented if the right measures are put in place to reduce the frequency of such accidents or eliminate them completely if possible.

Here are some workplace accident prevention tips:

Take Precautions against Blood-Borne Pathogens

While discharging their duties, health-care workers may come into contact with bodily fluids. This increases their exposure to blood-borne pathogens that may weaken their immunity and expose them to a series of ailments.

Health-care providers can minimize their exposure to such ailments by taking necessary measures such as wearing protective gear. Safety goggles, gowns, face shields and gloves help them to avoid coming into direct contact with potentially contaminated fluids.

Teach Important Safety Policies

The medical facility should provide staff, patients and others with information about important safety policies.

Have a Safety Compliance Plan

There is a huge difference between having a safety plan in place and having people comply with it. Such plans not only make it easier for safety plans to be followed but also help to promote positive treatment outcomes in addition to ensuring the safety of both the medical team and others.

Teach Patients Safety Information

It is important that patients are kept in the loop to assist the medical centers to succeed at their efforts to make their facilities secure and safe. Always explain the importance of staying safe. Make it a habit to consistently reiterate safety protocol and procedures as appropriate, to ensure patients stay in the know.

Safety and Health Management System

Care providers should create guidelines that help ensure the safety of health workers and patients.

Use Protective Equipment

To prevent accidents and infections, medical care staff should always use personal protective equipment such as masks, gloves and scrubs.

It is imperative that health-care workers are aware of the potential harms in different departments and use the most appropriate protective equipment to minimize danger.

High-quality masks are a necessity for medical workers attending to patients suffering from infectious diseases, while laundry workers need stronger gloves that can serve as protective gear against needles and other sharp objects that could be concealed in clothing, for example.

Report Hazards Immediately

While other industries may be content with just wiping off spills and leaks, bodily fluids such as blood may contain disease-transmitting bacteria. Wiping such fluids off won't be sufficient to eliminate the potential danger in them. More proactive measures must be taken, and protocols must be developed (and followed) to that effect.

Chapter Four: Medical Terminology

Your CMA examination will test your understanding of medical terminology. As a professional in the medical field, knowledge of medical terminology opens the door for effective communication with your colleagues, doctors and patients alike.

Thorough knowledge of medical terminology includes root words, prefixes and suffixes.

Root Words

A root word is a part of a word that provides basic meaning.

Prefixes

Prefixes are added to the beginning of a word to give the word a different meaning.

The following are some common medical prefixes, their meanings and possible usages in sentences:

Arthro-: When referring to bone joints, *arthro-* is the appropriate prefix. An example of the use of arthro- as a prefix is arthroscopic.

Bi-: *Bi-* means twice or double. An example of the use of bi- as a prefix is bicep.

Colpo-: Words related to the vagina have the *colpo-* prefix. It is from a Greek word, "kolpos," that means a cleft, fold or hollow. Colpopexy, colporrhaphy and colpocele are among the list of words with the prefix.

Extro/extra-: *Extro-* or *extra-* mean beyond or outside of. Extrovert, extrospection and extrude are some examples of such words.

Ferri-: *Ferri-* connotes iron. An example of a word using the prefix is ferric.

Gastr-: Conditions that are related to the stomach have the *gastr-* prefix. Some examples are gastronomy, gastropod and gastronome.

Hist-: Words and medical terms that are associated with tissue have *hist-* as the prefix. An example of a word using the prefix is histamine.

Intra-: *Intra-* means inside or within. Intravenous is one word that uses the prefix.

Kerat-: Cornea-related words usually have *kerat* as prefix. An example of a word using the prefix is keratolysis.

Lacto-: *Lacto-* means milk. An example of the prefix in a word is lactorrhea.

Lapar-: *Lapar* is a prefix associated with the abdomen or abdomen wall. Examples of words which use the prefix include laparocolostomy and laparectomy.

Mast-: *Mast-* is a prefix used for breast-related words. An example of a word using the prefix is mastectomy.

Melan-: *Melan-* means black. Melanin is one word that uses this prefix.

Micro-: *Micro-* means tiny or small. Microorganism is one word that uses the prefix.

Myo-: Ailments that are associated with the muscle tissue are easily identified by the *myo-* prefix. Myoglobin, myocyte, myotonia and myocarditis are some examples of such words.

Oophor: *Oophor-* is a prefix for ovary-related terms. Words that use this prefix include oophoroplasty, oophorrhagia and oophoroplasty.

Osseo-: *Osseo-* is specifically used as a prefix for bones. Osseocartilaginous is an example of a word that uses the prefix.

Pan-: *Pan-* means all or entire. An example of a word using the prefix is panimmunity.

Rhino-: This prefix is generally used to describe a medical condition that affects the nose. Examples include rhinocele, rhinocephaly and rhinogenous.

Ultra-: *Ultra-* mean excesses. Ultrasound and ultramodern are two examples of words with this prefix.

Suffixes

Medical suffixes are added to the end of root words to make their meanings clearer. They are most often used in the medical field in reference to operations, ailments, medical procedures and medications.

Some common medical suffixes are:

-ectasis: *-ectasis* is a suffix used for a wide range of health problems that are caused by the dilation of a body's hollow organ. Some typical examples of medical conditions that contain the suffix are bronchiectasis, esophagectasis and pyopyelectasis.

-gnosis: *-gnosis* means "knowledge," as in knowledge of a certain disease, for instance. Some common medical problems with the *-gnosis* suffix are lalognosis, barognosis, topognosis and autognosis.

-itis: Inflammation of any part of the body is expressed using the *-itis* suffix. Common examples are appendicitis, arthritis and bronchitis.

-pepsia: *-pepsia* is a suffix used for medical terms that express persistent pain in someone's upper abdomen, a health condition that may arise as a result of indigestion or problems associated with the digestive tract. Dyspepsia is an example of a word using the suffix.

Medical Specialties

Although medical practitioners are generally called doctors, there are hundreds of specialties a doctor may choose to specialize in.

Some common medical specialties are:

Anesthesiologists: These are medical doctors who specialize in numbing pain during childbirth, surgery or other painful procedures. They administer the appropriate dosage of the right drug to make the procedure less painful for patients. Anesthesiologists also monitor a patient's vital signs after administering anesthesia.

Cardiologists: Cardiologists treat ailments that are associated with blood vessels and the heart. They specialize in treating things such as heart attacks, irregular heartbeat and high blood pressure.

Dermatologists: Dermatologists handle health problems associated with the hair, skin and nails. Their job description includes treating inflammatory diseases affecting the skin, skin cancer and other infectious diseases common to the skin.

Endocrinologists: Endocrinologists address hormonal and metabolic disorders. They treat health problems such as thyroid problems, diabetes, calcium disorders, infertility and bone disorders.

Gastroenterologists: Gastroenterologists specialize in the digestive system. They treat diarrhea, abdominal pain, jaundice, ulcers, pancreatitis and cancers of the digestive organs, among many other conditions.

Geriatric Medicine Specialists: Geriatric medicine specialists attend to the medical needs of the elderly. They can work in an array of establishments such as doctors' offices, patients' homes, assisted-living centers, nursing homes and hospitals, where they treat a series of ailments specific to the elderly.

Hematologists: Hematologists treat diseases of the spleen, blood and lymph glands. Anemia, sickle cell disease, leukemia, hemophilia and anemia are some health conditions these specialists treat.

Immunologists/allergists: These professionals specialize in treating food allergies, asthma, insect sting allergies, eczema and other related immune system disorders.

Infectious Disease Specialists: These medical professionals diagnose and treat infectious diseases such as pneumonia, HIV/AIDS, Lyme disease and tuberculosis.

Internists: Internists are physicians who are primarily concerned with treating diseases affecting the internal organs. They treat diseases of the kidneys, heart, digestive system, joints, vascular system and respiratory system.

Medical Geneticists: Sometimes, parents pass hereditary disorders down to their children. Medical geneticists diagnose and treat such disorders and thus prevent them from having a permanent negative impact on the children's lives.

Neurologists: These physicians focus primarily on treating issues relating to the nervous system. They treat diseases of the peripheral nerves, brain, autonomic nervous system, spinal cord and blood vessels. Neurologists also treat people who suffer from Alzheimer's disease, strokes and seizure disorders.

Obstetrics/Gynecologists: These are specialists who deal with the female reproductive system. The profession covers an array of care that includes gynecologic care, primary health-care for women, oncology and when necessary, surgical operations. Gynecologic oncology, reconstructive surgery, reproductive endocrinology, female pelvic medicine and infertility are some areas OB-GYNs specialize in.

Ophthalmologists: Ophthalmologists provide medical care for the eyes. This may sometimes involve performing surgical operations. Some of the ailments they treat include diabetic retinopathy and strabismus.

Otolaryngologists: Medical disorders in the nose, ears, sinuses and throat are treated by these medical professionals. They also attend to health challenges in the neck, head and respiratory system. Their job descriptions include plastic and reconstructive surgery on the neck and the head to correct anomalies.

Pathologists: Pathologists diagnose and monitor diseases through clinical lab tests and microscopic examinations that allow them to identify the major causes of diseases and understand their nature.

Pediatricians: Pediatricians specialize in diagnosing and treating people from infancy to adolescence. Diseases common to infants such as allergies, asthma and croup are the domain of these experts. While they can treat a series of ailments, pediatricians may specialize in adolescent medicine, pediatric cardiology, pediatric endocrinology and pediatric infectious disease, among others.

Plastic Surgeons: Plastic surgeons specialize in repairing injured parts of the body, such as the face, skin, breasts and hands. They also perform plastic surgeries for cosmetic reasons.

Psychiatrists: Psychiatrists are trained to understand the connections between people's emotion, their genetics and mental illness. Community psychiatry, addiction psychiatry and forensic psychiatry are some of the subspecialties within this medical profession.

Surgical Procedures

There are different types of surgical procedures for different ailments. Some of the most common surgical procedures and their functions are:

Abdominoplasty: This surgical procedure is also known as a tummy tuck. It is a cosmetic surgery performed specifically for altering the abdomen's shape. An abdominoplasty is done to correct some obesity-triggered medical abnormalities, to fix defects in the abdomen or to correct health challenges that may arise after surgery or disease.

Amputation: Amputation is a surgical procedure that involves the removal of a patient's limb. This may be done to prevent an infection from spreading to the entire body, potentially killing the patient.

Appendectomy: This surgical procedure removes an inflamed or infected appendix. An appendectomy is otherwise referred to as an appendicectomy.

Breast Augmentation or Implants: During the surgical procedure, silicone shells are implanted under the muscles of the breasts or under the breasts themselves. This can be done to enlarge the breasts or as part of reconstructive surgery.

Gastric Bypass Surgery: This surgical operation decreases the stomach's size, helping obese individuals to lose weight.

Diseases and Pathologies

Medical professionals diagnose and treat an array of medical conditions, including:

Alopecia Areata: This medical problem attacks the hair follicles. Since these follicles are responsible for hair growth, the damage results in hair falling out.

Arthritis: Arthritis is an umbrella term for all diseases that cause discomfort in the joints. Its relatives are rheumatic diseases that affect not only the joints but may affect the bones, ligaments, muscles and tendons too.

Autoinflammatory Diseases: This type of ailment causes the accidental attack of the body by the immune cells. The attack can cause a wide range of health problems that include joint swelling, fever and other medical conditions.

Bursitis: Bursitis is a medical condition that is characterized by pain and swelling in some parts of the body, especially the bones and muscles.

Epidermolysis Bullosa: A group of diseases that trigger the development of painful blisters on the skin is called epidermolysis bullosa. While the blisters are naturally painful, they become particularly problematic if they are infected.

Gout: When crystals of uric acid build up in the joints, it results in a medical condition known as gout. This arthritis-like medical problem causes stiff joints that are usually painful.

Hidradenitis Suppurativa (HS): Another name for this ailment is acne inversa. It is a noncontagious and chronic inflammatory health problem with boils or pimple-like bumps as symptoms. It can attack both beneath the skin and above it.

Juvenile Arthritis: Juvenile arthritis occurs when a young child's joints are inflamed. The painful medical condition hampers movement.

Lichen Sclerosus: This health problem is generally characterized by white patches or spots in the anal areas or on the genitals. Nevertheless, it can also be found somewhere else on the victim's body. Other symptoms are pain, itching and bleeding.

Osteoarthritis: This is a painful health problem. Someone with this ailment will suffer damage to the tissues that cover the bones, especially at the ends. Thus, the bones will rub together. This will result in painful swelling. Individuals with osteoarthritis usually lose the ability to move.

Osteogenesis imperfecta: Otherwise known as brittle bone disease, this genetic ailment weakens the bones so that they break easily.

Paget's Disease of Bone: Paget's is a medical problem that affects bones. A bone will grow excessively large and weak. The disease is not limited to a specific bone in the body.

Pemphigus: While many ailments result in a weakened immune system, pemphigus causes the immune system to attack the skin's surface by damaging healthy cells found on top of the skin. This results in painful blisters.

Psoriatic Arthritis: This condition only affects people with psoriasis. These people have scaly white and red patches that create room for the ailment. Psoriatic arthritis affects parts of the joints and body where bone and tissues are attached together.

Rheumatoid Arthritis: Rheumatoid arthritis is a disease that can affect multiple joints simultaneously. Swelling, pain and stiffness are some of the common symptoms of the ailment. The sufferer may also experience unusual fever and tiredness.

Rosacea: Rosacea is a long-term medical ailment that causes pimples and reddened skin. It mostly affects the face and can also trigger eye problems and thicken the skin too.

Spinal Stenosis: The spine has a specific size and width. When the spine becomes unusually narrow, it results in a medical condition known as spinal stenosis. As the spine becomes narrow, more pressure is put on the nerves and spinal cord. The excessive pressure on these body parts may cause serious pain.

Sports Injuries: Sports injuries are classified into chronic and acute, depending on the duration and severity of the injury.

Tendinitis: This medical condition is known for causing pain and swelling in a joint. The condition usually arises when a tendon is repeatedly injured. Tendons are the part of the joint responsible for connecting the bones and muscles.

Vitiligo: This is a disorder that affects the skin. It causes some patches of the skin to gradually become white. The condition is triggered as a result of the destruction of the color-producing cells in a patient's skin.

Medical Abbreviations

You should be familiar with some common medical abbreviations used in the medical field. This is a short list of some of these abbreviations:

ACL: An anterior cruciate ligament is commonly known as a knee injury. Someone with ACL usually has a sprained or torn ligament.

ANED: ANED stands for alive, no evidence of disease. It is used in reference to a patient brought to a medical facility alive, without any traces of evidence of any disease.

ARDS: ARDS means acute respiratory distress syndrome. As the name implies, this is a medical condition that is characterized by respiratory failure. Its symptoms include shortness of breath, rapid breathing and skin discoloration.

ASCVD: ASCVD is atherosclerotic cardiovascular disease. This is a result of the buildup of harmful plaque in the walls of the arteries. Peripheral artery disease and coronary heart disease are some examples of ASCVD. It also covers aortic atherosclerotic diseases such as abdominal aortic aneurysms and descending thoracic aneurysms.

BSO: A bilateral salpingo-oophorectomy involves the removal of the fallopian tubes and the ovaries. It is usually a part of what is medically known as an abdominal hysterectomy.

CABG: CABG stands for coronary artery bypass graft. It refers to a form of surgical operation that is performed on the heart.

DOE: DOE means dyspnea on exertion. It is a medical term for shortness of breath that is triggered by nothing but excessive physical activity.

HPS: HPS is a contagious and infectious disease known as hantavirus pulmonary syndrome. The major carriers of the deadly disease are rats who transmit the ailment to unsuspecting victims through contact with the animals or consuming foods contaminated with rodents' waste products.

IBD: Inflammatory bowel disease is a medical condition that affects the gastrointestinal tract. IBD is also an umbrella name for Crohn's disease and ulcerative colitis.

IDDM: IDDM stands for insulin-dependent diabetes mellitus. Another name for IDDM is type 1 diabetes. It is a form of diabetes that is more difficult to treat than the type 2 variant.

ICU: ICU is a common word in the medical industry. It means intensive care unit, a reference to a section of the hospital or any medical facility where patients with serious medical conditions that need urgent attention are attended to.

LCIS: LCIS means lobular carcinoma in situ. It is an abbreviation for a particular type of cancer.

MTBI: A mild traumatic brain injury is commonly referred to as a concussion. MTBI is usually triggered by either violent shaking of the head or the entire body. Another causative factor is a deadly blow to the head. MBTI can cause headaches, fatigue, depression, anxiety, irritability and impaired cognitive function.

PE: A pulmonary embolism is a medical condition wherein blood clots in the lungs. This may cause permanent damage to the patient's health and threaten his/her life.

PRN: PRN means "as needed." It is a reference to the need for a medical procedure that is only done when there are no alternatives.

These are some common medical suffixes, prefixes and medical terminology that you should ensure you are familiar with.

Chapter Five: Establish Patient Medical Records

Medical records are documents that contain information about patients in a medical facility. Such records contain information such as each patient's age, medical history and other important information that may prove useful in treating the person.

Complete medical records may include any of the following:

Discharge Summary: Discharging patients from medical facilities is one of the regular responsibilities of health workers. Documenting the discharging process is important too. That is where a discharge summary comes in handy.
This clinical report is usually prepared by a professional health-care provider at the completion of a patient's stay in the medical facility. This important document sometimes bridges the communication gap between doctors and other after-care providers. Some information contained in the discharge summary are patient name, date of birth, unique identification number, telephone number, gender, ethnicity, address and next of kin or emergency contact. The discharge summary also contains hospital details such as the discharging consultant, date and time of both the admission and discharge as well as discharge destination.

Diagnostic Test: In the medical field, a diagnostic test is any form of approach used by the medical team for the purpose of gathering clinical information that will assist them to make informed decisions such as diagnoses. Pregnancy tests, X-rays, medical histories and biopsies are some important diagnostic tests that provide medical practitioners with the information they need for further treatment.

Clinical Correspondence: Clinical correspondence refers to information about a specific patient sent by a health organization or a doctor. It also refers to information received by a medical practitioner or an organization.

Operative Note: This is also known as an operative report. It is a report about a patient written in his/her medical record after a surgical operation. In the note, the surgical procedure is documented to give insight into the entire process and provide information about the surgery to the medical staff whenever they need such information. In the note is the preoperative diagnosis and postoperative diagnosis. The patient's condition after the surgery is also documented.

Other information you can find in the note is the technical procedure used for the surgical operation, the removed specimens, estimated volume of blood loss and the names of both the primary and assistant surgeons.

Flow Sheet: A flow sheet is a document containing important data about a patient's condition. This document is usually kept in the patient's chart, where it can be referenced to provide information about the care given to the patient.

Flow sheets help medical practitioners to record patient's health vitals and track such information when necessary. The patient's pain severity and hunger level may be captured in the flow sheet as well.

Flow sheets enable practitioners to flag abnormal values as well as plot data that may enable them to see changes that are happening in their patients. They act as a working note that allows health-care professionals to record a chronological account of each patient's illnesses. Thus, clinicians can use the information for more important treatments in the future.

Clinic Progress Note: The progress notes are important components of a patient's medical record. This sheet serves as a platform for health-care professionals to record the clinical status of a patient. The sheet covers important information about the patient, especially during hospitalization. The care and treatment given are also documented because they are integral to the treatment process.

Charting Systems

In the medical world, there are two charting systems that assist medical practitioners in making the best use of patients' medical records. These are:

Source-Oriented Medical Record (SOMR)

The Source-Oriented Medical Record is used for updating medical records.

SOMR is used in charts that are divided into sections that include:

Progress Notes: As the name suggests, these notes contain important information about a patient's progress while receiving treatment in a hospital. The record details the patient's progress, irrespective of whether the patient is receiving outpatient care or is hospitalized in the medical facility.

History and Physical: History and Physical is an important reference document which contains information such as the patient's medical history and results of examinations done when the patient was to be admitted.

Diagnostic Testing: This refers to any technique used by a medical facility to gather clinical information from patients. Such information is used for diagnoses or clinical decisions. Some examples of diagnostic tests are medical histories, X-rays, pregnancy tests and biopsies.

Problem-Oriented Medical Record (POMR)

The Problem-Oriented Medical Record is a method used in the medical field for recording important data about a patient's health status.

POMR addresses several issues and offers the following benefits:

- It enables medical teams to document chronic illnesses with ease.
- When a patient is being attended to by at least two physicians, POMR helps avoid confusion.
- It also helps when a patient is treated for multiple illnesses simultaneously.
- Patients with such records have better knowledge of themselves and their health. They are also more likely to handle their health better than patients without such records.

Dr. Lawrence Weed, the creator of this system, emphasized some of the POMR's useful attributes:

It can be quite challenging to manage chronic illnesses. Most often, multiple interventions are required to treat such ailments. This may require making adjustments to existing plans over time in order to effectively cure the ailment. This requires medical experts to track their interventions and physiological variables over time. POMR makes this easier to do.

Some patients with complex medical conditions require constant medical care. Examples are patients with multimorbidity and other chronic ailments. Multiple clinicians must attend to these patients' medical needs. For efficient performance, their activities must be coordinated over time. When a medical challenge arises, individualized health care is best. It is easier to track such care through POMR.

It is important that patients are aware of their own medical needs. This will trigger a sense of commitment and participation, an essential tool for treatment as patients then play a part in their recovery.

Medical data must be charted to enable health-care providers to provide their patients with individualized medical attention.

The importance of medical records can't be overemphasized. Thus, it is imperative that medical workers find convenient ways to get the best out of these records.

Chapter Six: Scheduling Appointments

Appointment scheduling can have a huge impact on any medical provider's success. Ensuring that patients are attended to at the right time can help to maximize resources efficiently.

When a physician is overwhelmed with work, it is a medical assistant's responsibility to schedule appointments. Thus, you determine who visits the physician, when and for how long.

Factors to Consider when Scheduling a Medical Appointment

You can schedule successful medical appointments if you consider the following factors:

Physician Preferences: What appointment method does the physician favor? Does the physician prefer to have patients waiting, or can he/she see a couple of patients at a time? Should you schedule a break at regular intervals or in between patients? Don't forget that the doctor may have other tasks to attend to during the day. Find a time for such tasks when making the appointments. Other tasks you may factor in include chart examinations and phone calls.

Available Facilities: The available facilities should be considered too. It is pointless to schedule multiple appointments for the same procedure if existing facilities are insufficient to accommodate such procedures simultaneously. So, be aware of the facilities that are available for a procedure and the number of such procedures that can be attended to at a time.

Patients' Needs: When will patients be available for such appointments? This involves considering patients' work schedules. For instance, while some patients may be able to come in during the week, some may not be able to be seen until the weekend. How long will it take patients to get to the medical facility? What about the patients' ages? Can they make a long trip to the doctor or not?

You should have a comprehensive knowledge of patients' needs and build your appointments around them.

Duration of the Visit: What type of visit are you considering? Remember that a minor exam or checkup shouldn't be compared with a surgery that obviously will require more time and attention. Then, consider how much time an appointment will require from the doctor.

Types of Appointments

There are different types of appointment scheduling. Some of these are:

Scheduled Appointments: The scheduled appointment considers the time needed for a procedure before booking appointments for patients. As a medical assistant, your knowledge of the different procedures and their duration will determine the time allocated for each visit.

Open Office Hours: With this type of scheduling, patients are allowed to see the doctor in order of their arrival. This appointment type completely eliminates appointment cancelation or other problematic situations where patients arrive for appointments far behind schedule.

With this appointment schedule type, the physician may be less busy some hours of the day and may have a long list of waiting patients to attend to at some other hours.

Advanced Scheduling: This scheduling appointment type involves booking an appointment prior to when a person needs to see the doctor later on in the year, for example. As a medical assistant, it is your responsibility to remind patients of their advanced appointments. In some cases, some physicians require that they receive 24 hours' notice if the patient wants to cancel the appointment. This enables a doctor to fill the appointment time rather than waste time and resources.

Flexible Office Hours: Some patients may find it difficult to meet appointments made during fixed office hours. Using flexible office hours, you can book appointments for such patients on weekend hours or evenings.

Wave Scheduling: Wave scheduling is a scheduling type that offers some flexibility. It is a method that involves planning a specific number of appointments within a specific period of time. For instance, while some scheduling types involve assigning a fixed time to each appointment, say 10 minutes, wave scheduling involves booking six appointments within an hour. Thus, the appointments are attended to on a first-come, first-served basis.

Appointment Scheduling Guidelines

Below are some practical tips that can help you to make effective appointment schedules:

Prioritize the Appointments: Patients' needs are diverse. Thus, the degree of time needed to attend to each person will differ as well. Patients also need different levels of care. When scheduling a patient's appointment, it is important that you consider all these factors to enable you to make the right decision.

If you have patients who require little time, you may be able to help them over the phone. Alternatively, schedule their appointments at a time that won't interfere with other patients who obviously need more attention.

Use Appointment Reminders: Appointment reminders are designed to remind you of existing appointments. By using a software system, you are more likely to keep up with your appointments.

Use a Waiting List: Sometimes, it may be quite frustrating to deal with last-minute cancellations, especially if you have nothing to fill the vacuum. You can spare yourself this problem by creating a patient waiting list. When cancelations occur, you can easily replace the unavailable patient with someone else from the list. Having such a list on hand can save you a lot of time and resources.

Some special circumstances are also considered when booking appointments. These are:

Rescheduling Canceled Appointment: When the need to reschedule a canceled appointment arises, remove the first appointment. Then, reschedule the appointment to avoid a conflict of appointments.

Late Patients: You will sometimes come across habitually late patients. You can handle such cases by scheduling such patients for the last appointment of the day. You can also ask such patients to arrive before their actual appointment time. This will make up for their lateness. However, if after all is said and done, the patient still comes in late, the physician isn't under obligation to attend them.

Physician Referrals: Physician referrals shouldn't be ignored when planning appointments. You should always leave enough room to accommodate such requests from other medical personnel.

Emergency Calls: Responding to emergencies is part of every physician's job description. When patients need to see a physician urgently, you must be able to rise to the occasion. However, it is imperative that you screen seemingly urgent calls and identify conditions that actually demand urgent medical attention.

Appointment Protocols

- **Tickler File:** A ticker file is otherwise known as a 43 Folder System. It is a collection of file folders with some specific days. The file is organized so that time-sensitive documents can easily be retrieved for use since the primary filing factor is date. Such documents are used for a wide range of time-based activities such as pending bills, meeting information and other things such as appointment scheduling.

The folder for each day is retrieved to enable the physician to act on the appointments for the day. Recently, the file has been automated through software programs that are designed to automatically set a reminder about the appointments for the day. When you feed the automated file the necessary information, the physician will get a timely reminder every day.

- **Physician Delay:** Doctor delay is another issue with booking appointments. A doctor may be quite busy, and taking on new medical cases may not be advisable at a given moment. When booking appointments, create room for such unexpected delays so that some patients won't be waiting anxiously while the doctor has more free time than expected.

You can enhance your productivity by ensuring that patients are well scheduled. Aside from helping a physician, it helps to keep patients from having to wait for extended periods of time.

Chapter Seven: Anatomy & Physiology

The body is made primarily of five vital organs. These are the kidneys, brain, liver, heart and lungs.

Kidneys

On either side of the human spine is a kidney, a bean-shaped internal body organ. It is located behind the belly and below the ribs. Each kidney is about five inches long and is approximately the size of a large fist.

The kidneys are designed to filter blood. During filtration, they ensure that the body's fluid is balanced in addition to removing waste. They also keep the body's electrolytes at the right levels.

Each kidney has about one million nephrons (tiny filters). The nephrons support the kidneys and ensure they function at maximum capacity.

Kidney failure may occur when the kidneys are denied blood. This may lead to partial or total death of the affected kidney.

The main functions of the kidneys are:

- Acid-base balance
- Ensuring water balance
- Controlling electrolyte balance
- Blood pressure control
- Removing waste products and toxins from the body

Brain

The human brain is undoubtedly the most complex body part. It is the control center of the entire body, thanks to its over 100 billion nerves that use synapses for communication.

The brain is responsible for sending and receiving signals to every other part of the body through secreted hormones and the nervous system.

The brain is also responsible for feelings, thoughts and memory storage.

Anatomy of the Human Brain

The cerebrum forms the largest part of the brain. The brain is comprised of the forebrain, midbrain and hindbrain. Each part is made up of ventricles, which are cavities filled with fluid.

Some areas of the brain that perform important functions are:

The Cortex: The outermost layer of this important organ is the cortex. The cortex is the starting point for voluntary movements and thinking.

The Brainstem: This part of the brain, located at the base, is responsible for controlling basic functions such as sleep and breathing.

The Cerebellum: The cerebellum is also located at the brain's base. Without this essential brain part, balance and coordination are impossible.

The Basal Ganglia: In the center of the brain is located a cluster of structures that form the basal ganglia. It is responsible for coordinating messages between the brain and other areas.

The brain is divided into the following lobes:

Frontal Lobes: An individual's problem-solving abilities are controlled by the frontal lobes. They are also responsible for people's motor function and judgment.

Occipital Lobes: The occipital lobes regulate the brain's ability to process things, functioning as its visual processing system.

Temporal Lobes: These are designed to control each individual's hearing and memory.

Parietal Lobe: This part of the brain interprets sensory information.

Liver

The liver is another large organ of the body. It is located on the belly's right side. Serving as protection for the liver is the rib cage.

The liver is divided into the left and right lobes. Under the liver are the pancreas, gallbladder and the intestines. These organs work together with the liver to perform multiple functions such as food digestion, absorption and processing.

Blood filtration is the liver's primary responsibility. It filters blood from the digestive tract before the blood is transported to every other part of the body.

It also serves as a detoxification and metabolic agent for chemicals and drugs to enable the body to assimilate and use them.

As it performs its functions, the liver secretes bile that eventually ends up in the intestines. This greenish-brown and bitter fluid is stored in the gall bladder and it aids digestion. It also provides proteins needed in the body for blood clotting and other important bodily functions.

Heart

The heart is the organ responsible for circulating blood throughout the body. In the human body, the circulatory system revolves around the heart. The four-chambered double pump is between the two lungs; they ensure that the body receives the needed amount of blood for proper functioning.

The heart is roughly the same shape and size as a closed fist. Two-third of its entire mass is located towards the left of the heart.

The heart wall is formed by three layers. The epicardium is the outer layer and the middle is the myocardium. The inner layer is made up of the endocardium.

The heart's internal cavity is divided into four layers. These are the right atrium, left atrium, right ventricle and left ventricle.

The thin-walled chambers of the heart are the atria. The veins pass blood to the atria, while the thick-walled chambers known as the ventricles are the channels through which blood is pumped out of the heart.

You will notice some differences in the thickness of the heart's chamber walls. The differences are caused by the different amounts of myocardium in the heart, a reflection of the amount of force that must be generated by each chamber.

Deoxygenated blood is passed to the right atrium from the systemic veins, while the pulmonary veins pass oxygenated blood to the left atrium.

Lungs

The lungs are located on either side of the thorax or chest. Lungs are spongy and filled with air. They are also soft and elastic. Healthy lungs float in water and when squeezed, they will crackle.

The windpipe or trachea transports inhaled air through the bronchi or tubular branches into the lungs. Then, the tubular branches divide into bronchioles.

Microscopic air sacs are usually the final destinations for the bronchioles. These air sacs are known as alveoli. In these sacs, the blood absorbs oxygen from the air, while carbon dioxide moves to the alveoli from the blood before it is eventually exhaled through the alveoli.

The primary responsibilities of the lungs are adding oxygen to the blood and removing carbon dioxide from it.

The pleura is a thin tissue layer that covers the lungs and external part of the chest cavity.

Each lung is divided into lobes. A tissue fissure separates the lobes from one another.

There are three lobes in the right lung. The left lung has two lobes because it is bigger than the right lung. The asymmetrical shape of the heart is responsible for the differences in sizes of the pair of lungs.

Hundreds of lobes make up each lobe internally. The components of each of the lobules are a thin wall, a bronchiole, clusters of alveoli and affiliated branches.

While the lungs are primarily designed for respiratory activities, they also perform some other functions. Without them, we couldn't absorb and excrete substances such as alcohol and water. Pharmacologic agents are also absorbed with the assistance of the lungs.

The lungs also perform some metabolic functions. They are involved in the storage, degradation, storage and synthesis of a wide range of substances such as fibrin, surfactant, angiotensin, histamine, prostaglandins and other molecules.

If you are active, you only use about one-twentieth of the lung's gaseous-exchange surface. As your engagement in vigorous physical activity increases, the portion of the surface you use increases correspondingly.

Diseases of the Organs

The following are some diseases of the body's organs:

Liver

The liver is susceptible to the following medical conditions:

Cirrhosis: When the liver is damaged permanently, cirrhosis occurs. It is characterized by permanent scarring of the liver.

Gallstones: Gallstones can pose a serious risk to the liver. If a stone becomes stuck in the liver-draining bile duct, that may result in an infection.

Hemochromatosis: This ailment is triggered when iron is deposited in the liver. The deposited iron damages the liver. The iron is also deposited in other body parts, causing multiple health problems.

Hepatitis: Hepatitis is an inflammation of the liver. Three types of hepatitis viruses cause this medical condition: hepatitis A, hepatitis B and hepatitis C.
Other non-infectious causes of hepatitis are allergic reactions, heavy drinking, obesity and drugs.

Liver Failure: As the name implies, this ailment occurs when the liver is no longer functional. This may be triggered by an array of factors that include but are not limited to genetic diseases, infection and excessive alcohol consumption.

Heart

Some of the most common heart-related medical conditions are:

Arrhythmia: This medical condition is also known as dysrhythmia. It is an abnormal heart rhythm that occurs when the conduction of electrical impulses via the heart undergoes some changes. Some cases of this medical condition may be mild, while others are life-threatening.

Cardiomyopathy: This ailment affects the heart muscle. The muscle becomes abnormally thick, enlarged or stiff. This is in addition to other physical changes that make it difficult for the heart to perform its blood-pumping function.

Coronary Artery Disease: Coronary artery disease is caused by the accumulation of cholesterol plaque in the heart. Such accumulation usually results in the narrowing of the arteries that transport blood to the heart. The blocked arteries are always at risk of being completely blocked when the blood undergoes sudden clotting. Such a blockage is medically referred to as a heart attack.

Pericarditis: When the pericardium or lining of the heart is inflamed, it results in pericarditis. Some common causes of the heart problem include kidney failure, viral infections and autoimmune conditions.

Stable Angina Pectoris: When the coronary arteries are narrowed, this can result in discomfort or chest pain when they are exerted. As a result of the blockage, the heart is denied the extra oxygen it needs to carry out strenuous activities. That can have a huge negative impact on the heart.

The heart has four valves. If any of them develops a severe problem, congestive heart failure may result.

Lungs

The lungs can be affected by several medical conditions that include:

Asthma: Asthma is one of the most common lung ailments. It occurs as a result of the inflammation of the bronchi or the lungs' airways. This may result in wheezing and shortness of breath. Viral infections, allergies and air pollution are factors that may trigger this lung-related medical condition.

Bronchiectasis: An abnormal inflammation of the lungs' airways is the primary cause of bronchiectasis. It may also arise from how the bronchi are impacted. Either condition may cause bronchiectasis, especially after the lungs have been subjected to repeated infections. The ailment's main symptom is repeated coughing.

Chronic Obstructive Pulmonary Disease (COPD): COPD is a health problem that may be triggered by cigarette smoking, genetic conditions, infectious diseases and air pollution. When the lungs are damaged, they find it increasingly difficult to function at maximum capacity. This may increase breathing difficulty.

Cystic Fibrosis: This is a genetic condition that is characterized by difficulty in expelling mucus from the airways. The excess mucus leads to repeated cases of pneumonia and bronchitis. There is no cure for the condition.

Pleurisy: Pleurisy refers to the inflammation of the pleura, the lining of the lungs. A victim of this ailment will feel pain when inhaling. Infections, autoimmune conditions and pulmonary embolisms are some common causes of pleurisy.

Kidneys

A patient with malfunctioning kidneys is prone to the following medical conditions:

Acute Renal Failure: Commonly referred to as kidney failure, this medical condition is characterized by a sudden depreciation in the kidneys' functioning power. Severe cases may include kidney damage or a blockage of the urinary tract.

Nephrogenic Diabetes Insipidus: This medical condition occurs when the kidneys can no longer concentrate the urine. It is triggered by a drug reaction. Although this health problem may be mild, it can cause frequent urination and constant thirst.

Nephrotic Syndrome: When the kidneys are damaged, they contaminate the urine with large amounts of protein. This may trigger edema or leg swelling.

Papillary Necrosis: When severely damaged, the kidney tissues may break internally, thereby clogging the kidneys. If this condition is left untreated, it may result in papillary necrosis or total kidney failure.

Pyelonephritis: Pyelonephritis occurs when a bladder infection is left untreated. This may result in fever or back pain.

The Body Systems

The human body's operations are controlled by a series of systems. In this section, we will take a look at some of the systems, their functions and composition.

Urinary System

The body gets the energy it needs by taking nutrients from food. It changes the nutrients into energy. After taking the portion of the food it needs, the body leaves the rest as waste in the blood and bowels.

The urinary system's primary responsibility is to get rid of the urea or liquid waste. It also assists with keeping chemicals such as sodium and potassium and water in balance.

Urea production follows a simple process. When someone consumes protein-rich foods such as poultry and meat, they are broken down in the individual's body to form urea. The waste is subsequently transported to the kidneys through the blood. The urea and other waste are removed from the body as urine.

The urinary system is made of the urethra, kidneys, bladder and ureters.

Aside from waste product elimination from the body, the urinary system also regulates blood pressure. It supports erythropoietin production, a substance that works in the bone marrow to control red blood cell production.

The kidneys, vital urinary organs, support fluid conservation and acid-balance regulation too.

The functions of the major components of the urinary system are discussed below:

Kidneys: The kidneys are located in the middle of the back and below the ribs. They serve the following functions:

- They balance bodily fluids
- They remove medicines and waste products from the body
- They release the hormones needed for controlling the amount and volume of red blood cells produced in the body
- They release hormones that are necessary for blood pressure control
- They control phosphorus and calcium levels

Ureters: There are two ureters in the urinary system which transport urine to the bladder from the kidneys. They also eliminate urine from the bladder through the tightening and relaxing of the ureter walls' muscles. This results in urine elimination from the kidneys. The ureters empty small quantities of urine into the bladder every 10 to 15 seconds.

Urethra: This tube serves as the channel between the urine in the bladder and the outside world. The urine passes through the urethra on its way to the outside. The bladder receives signals from the brain to tighten and thereby squeeze and push the urine out. Simultaneously, the sphincter muscles receive further signals from the brain to relax and give the urine easy passage through the urethra. Urination is the end result of the signals received by these parts.

Bladder: The bladder is a hollow organ in the lower belly. The triangle-shaped organ stores urine due to the expansion and relaxation of its walls. The bladder's walls contract and flatten to allow room for urine to exit through the urethra. A healthy adult can store about two cups of urine in his or her bladder for up to five hours.

Nerves: These nerves are present in the bladder. They alert someone of the need to empty the bladder through urination.

Two Sphincter Muscles: These are circular muscles that prevent accidental leaking of the urine. They close around the bladder's opening to prevent urine from leaking out.

Reproductive System

The reproductive system performs four major functions. These are:

- Egg and sperm cell production
- Transportation and sustenance of the produced cells
- Nurturing of the developing offspring
- Hormone production

The Female Reproductive System

The female reproductive system performs a wide range of functions. The production of egg cells takes place in the female reproductive system.

The system also ensures the transportation of the ova to where fertilization will occur.

In the fallopian tubes, sperm fertilize the egg and allow it to move to the next stage, where the fertilized egg will be implanted into the uterus' walls. This is the beginning of pregnancy.

If for any reason, fertilization doesn't occur, the reproductive system will get rid of the eggs through menstruation, medically defined as the shedding of the uterine lining.

To keep the reproductive cycle going, the female reproductive system also produces female sex hormones.

The female reproductive system is divided into external reproductive organs and internal reproductive organs.

Internal Female Reproductive Organs

The internal reproductive organs are the uterus, vagina, ovaries and fallopian tubes. These organs perform different but related functions that make reproduction possible.

Vagina: This is a muscular and hollow tube extending from the opening of the vaginal to the uterus. The muscular walls enable it to contract and expand when necessary. To keep the vagina moist and protected, mucous membranes line its muscular walls.

To plays its role as a member of the reproductive system, the vagina performs these three different functions:

- Entrance for the penis during sexual intercourse
- Pathway for baby during childbirth
- Passage for blood during menstruation

The vagina's opening is covered by a thin tissue, the hymen. This differs from one woman to another. Hymens are most often broken during the first sexual experience, while some women have theirs broken before their first sexual encounter.

If it is not yet broken before the first coitus, the hymen may bleed a little during intercourse, usually accompanied by a little pain.

Uterus: The uterus is commonly known as the womb. It has muscular walls and a thick lining. The muscles can contract and expand, allowing a growing fetus enough space to grow without harm. They are also used for pushing the baby out during childbirth. In a non-pregnant woman, the uterus is about two inches wide and three inches long (five centimeters wide and 7.5 centimeters long.)

Fallopian Tubes: The ovaries are connected to the uterus through the fallopian tubes. The tubes are narrow and attached to the uterus' upper part. They are the channels of transportation for the ova when moving to the uterus from the ovaries.

Fertilization occurs in the fallopian tubes. After their fertilization, the eggs will move to the uterus, where they are implanted into the uterine wall's lining.

Ovaries: These are oval-shaped organs located at either side of the uterus. They are primarily designed for producing, storing and releasing eggs through ovulation into the fallopian tubes. Aside from egg production, they produce hormones as well.

External Female Reproductive Organs

The external organs of the female reproductive system are:

Labia Minora: The small labia are about two inches wide. They are inside the labia majora, where they surround the urethra that transports urine from the bladder away from the body and the vagina.

Labia Majora: The labia majora protect the external reproductive organs by enclosing them. They are fleshy and large and compare to the male scrotum due to their size and shape. This external organ contains oil-secreting glands and sweat. In adult females, they are usually covered with hair.

Clitoris: The clitoris is the meeting point for the two labia minora. It is a small but very sensitive part of the female reproductive organs that protrudes in a manner that draws comparisons between it and a penis.

The prepuce, a fold of skin, covers the clitoris; it can be compared to the penis' foreskin. When fully stimulated, the clitoris becomes erect like a penis.

Male Reproductive System

The male reproductive system serves the same purpose as the female reproductive system: procreation. Thus, it consists of special organs that are specifically designed for reproduction.

The male reproductive organs include:

The Accessory Glands: The accessory glands include the prostate gland and the seminal vesicles. These organs provide the fluids needed by the duct system for lubrication. The sperm is also nourished with the fluids.

The urethra is the channel through which sperm is transported outside of the male body into the vagina during sexual intercourse.

The Duct System: The vas deferens and the epididymis make up the duct system. These organs transport sperm.

Testicles: In adult males, the testicles are oval-shaped reproductive organs. They produce millions of sperm cells and store them.

The Penis: The external part of the penis consists of spongy tissue with contraction and expansion abilities.

The penis has two major parts—the glans and the shaft. The main penis part is the shaft, while the glans, otherwise called the head, is the tip. The glans has a small opening or slit at its end. The opening is used for urination and ejaculation.

The male reproductive system performs some functions that include:

a. Semen production
b. The release of semen into a female's reproductive system during sexual intercourse
c. The production of sex hormones, an indication that an adult man has become sexually active at puberty

An adult male at puberty produces millions of sperm cells daily. These are tiny cells about 0.05 millimeters long. These sperm develop in the seminiferous tubules located in the testicles.

Each male has seminiferous tubules at birth. They contain some round cells. When a male reaches puberty, testosterone and other related hormones trigger the transformation of the simple cells in the tubules into sperm cells.

The cells undergo division and transformation until each assumes a tadpole-like structure with a short tail and a head. Safely kept in the head is genetic material.

The sperm will subsequently relocate to the epididymis, where they will undergo complete development.

After they have developed completely, the sperm are transported to the vas deferens or sperm duct. Here, the prostate gland and the seminal vesicles produce seminal fluid. During sexual stimulation of a male, the seminal fluid will form semen by mixing with sperm.

The stimulation also leads to the hardening of the once limp penis, a sign of sexual excitement. The tissues in the penis will subsequently be filled with blood that makes it erect and stiff.

Thus, during sexual intercourse, it is easier for the erect penis to be inserted into the vagina.

Sexual intercourse increases the stimulation of the erect penis. This forces the contraction of the muscles surrounding the reproductive organs. As the contraction continues, the semen is forced out through the urethra and the duct system.

Finally, ejaculation occurs when the semen enters the female reproductive organ, the vagina, through the urethra. With each ejaculation, some 500 million sperm are released.

Diseases of the Body Systems

Some medical conditions that are common to some of the body systems are discussed below:

Urinary System

Some diseases that are common to the urinary system include:

Incontinence: This medical condition is common to the urinary system. Victims of this ailment usually have the urge to urinate frequently; urine leakage is another common symptom, especially in women.

Male victims usually struggle with incomplete bladder emptying due to the enlargement of the victim's prostate, thereby obstructing bladder emptying. Frequent urination at night is a common problem.

Urinary Tract Infections (UTIs): This occurs in the urinary system when the urinary tract is affected by bacteria. The bacteria can affect several organs such as the bladder, urethra and the kidneys. While this problem is more common in women, men are not immune to it. Over eight million people are affected by urinary tract infections, according to the American Urological Association.

Interstitial Cystitis (IC): Another name for this ailment that is common to the urinary system is painful bladder syndrome. The chronic bladder problem is common in women, causing the victim bladder pain and pressure. Pelvic pain is another common system, although the degree varies from one victim to another.
IC can result in bladder scarring as well as hamper the bladder's elasticity. A defect in the lining that protects the bladder is common to interstitial cystitis.

Reproductive System

These are some of the medical conditions that affect the reproductive system.

Ovarian Cancer: This form of cancer specifically affects the female reproductive system.

Menstrual Cramping: Females may experience severe menstrual cramping, known in the medical field as dysmenorrhea. The severe pain may occur before the period or during it. It may last for a day or a week.

Vaginal Yeast Infection: This is another disease of the reproductive system common in females. As the name implies, it is a disease of the vagina that can be traced to a yeast fungus. This condition can be treated easily with over-the-counter drugs.

Endometriosis: This condition affects the endometrium, the inside of the uterus. It gradually moves to the outside of the uterus and affects organs such as the bowels, ovaries and the tissue lining the victim's pelvis. When the endometrial tissue is trapped, it results in a painful medical condition.

Pelvic Inflammatory Disease: This generally refers to an infection that affects any of the female reproductive organs. This may include the ovaries and the uterus. The medical condition can be traced to sexually transmitted diseases (STDs) such as chlamydia and gonorrhea. Aside from pelvic inflammatory disease, STDs can also trigger infertility.

Prostate Cancer: Prostate cancer is a male reproductive system medical condition. It affects the small gland that produces the seminal fluid used for nourishing and transporting sperm. It is the most common disease that affects the male reproductive organs and can result in an array of medical conditions such as frequent urination, erectile dysfunction, bloodstained semen or urine, urination difficulty or a painful sensation during ejaculation or urination. It can be treated by radiation therapy, surgery and/or hormonal treatment.

Prostatitis: This is characterized by inflammation or swelling of the prostate gland. It can lead to difficult or painful ejaculation and urination. The disease affects almost half of all grown men at some point in their lives.

Erectile Dysfunction: Erectile dysfunction is a medical condition in which a man can't get an erection or is unable to sustain an erection for sexual intercourse. According to some medical experts, almost one out of every 10 males experience the chronic and untreatable form of this ailment. The medical condition can also trigger vascular disease and a host of neurological disorders such as trauma, multiple sclerosis and some psychological issues.

Conception

After ejaculations, millions of sperm swim from the vagina through the uterus and the cervix into the fallopian tube to meet the newly released egg. The egg needs just one sperm to fertilize it.

The fertilized egg, now referred to as a zygote, is made up of 46 chromosomes—23 chromosomes from the sperm and the other half from the egg. They combine to form a zygote.

The zygote undergoes repeated divisions as it grows in the uterus. Gradually, it matures, first into an embryo, and subsequently into a fetus, until it grows into a baby ready for delivery.

Chapter Eight: Infection Control

Infection control is a measure taken by medical experts, medical assistants inclusive, to prevent the spread of infections in the community, among medical staff and patients, as well as within health-care facilities.

It is your responsibility as a medical assistant to support every preventive measure put in place to protect facilities and people against infections.

Before we discuss how to prevent infections, let's take a look at some of the agents that pass infections from one person to another.

Infectious Agents

Infectious agents are carriers of infections from one person to another. The following are some of the common infectious agents and the infections they spread:

Viruses

Viruses are destructive microscopic organisms. They are known to infect plants, animals, bacteria and fungi.

Viruses are carriers of deadly diseases. In some cases, viral infections may not trigger any traceable reaction.

Viruses are made up of DNA or RNA. They are usually surrounded by a coat of lipids, proteins or glycoprotein, proof of their complexity. They are parasitic organisms, and that explains why they always thrive in the presence of a host, not otherwise.

Viruses top the list of the world's most abundant biological entity, and they usually transmit incurable but manageable diseases.

Viral infections are usually transmitted from one person to another. It is not unheard of for nursing mothers to transmit infections to their children during delivery or pregnancy.

These infections are transmitted through various channels that include:

- Saliva exchange during sneezing or coughing
- Physical touch
- Contaminated water or food
- Sexual contact
- Animals or insects

Another characteristic of viruses is their ability to live on inanimate objects for a specific period of time. Thus, if a healthy person touches a virus-infected item, the person runs the risk of contracting the virus through the object, commonly referred to as a fomite.

Herpes, rabies, Ebola and COVID-19 are some types of viral infections. Others are measles, hepatitis, dengue fever, HIV, hepatitis and polio.

Parasites

Parasites are living organisms whose existence depends on another living organism. They are mostly disease carriers and may undermine their host's health.

Some parasites gain entrance to the host's body through contaminated water or food, while others live on the host's hair or skin.

Most parasites are microscopic; they can't be seen with the naked eye.

Some examples of parasites are:

- Crab lice
- Protozoa
- Skin mites or scabies
- Stomach worms
- Giardiasis
- Hookworm

Bacteria

Bacteria are the hosts for deadly diseases such as bacterial pneumonia, diphtheria, tuberculosis and typhoid. They are also the carriers for deadly diseases such as cholera, plague and dysentery. Mycobacterium tuberculosis (TB), Yersinia pestis (bubonic plague), Treponema pallidum (syphilis), cholera, salmonella and tetanus are some bacteria-carrying medical conditions.

Fungi

Fungi are some of the most destructive infectious agents. These agents can grow in different types of environments. They are ubiquitous and transport several ailments from one person to another.

There are different types of fungi. Some are molds, yeasts and dimorphic yeast, a form of fungi whose behavior is determined by its environment. While it sometimes exists as a yeast under some conditions, it functions as mold in other conditions.

Dimorphic yeasts can live in humans and a wide range of environments where they can transfer evasive diseases that otherwise healthy humans are not immune to. Some examples are Blastomyces dermatitidis, Histoplasma capsulatum, Sporothrix schenckii, Coccidioides immitis and Paracoccidioides brasiliensis. These agents are otherwise known as endemic fungi.

Fungi are the cause of several diseases such as athlete's foot and ringworm. Mycoses, histoplasmosis, aspergillosis and coccidioidomycosis are some fungal diseases.

Modes of Infection Transmission

Infectious diseases are transmitted in several ways. Some of these modes of transmission are:

Indirect Contact

Infectious diseases can be transmitted when a healthy person comes in direct contact with the carrier.

This transmission type can further be divided into:

Droplet Spread: When someone infected sneezes or coughs, he/she may spray droplets of saliva. These droplets may transmit the infection into a healthy person that comes in contact with them.

Person-to-Person Contact: Person-to-person contact is the most common way that most infectious diseases are transmitted. When an infected person exchanges bodily fluids with a healthy person, he/she runs the risk of being infected. This is the primary transmission channel for STDs.

Coming into direct physical contact with the infected person through touching, kissing and hugging can also trigger infection transmission.

Direct Contact

Infection transmission through direct contact is referred to as contagious disease. These infections require physical contact with the infected person through the sharing of personal effects such as towels, socks and other clothing, especially if such items are not thoroughly washed before they are shared with others.

Human bites and sharing contaminated syringes are some other ways indirect person-to-person contact can occur, thereby triggering disease transmission.

Impetigo, athlete's foot, conjunctivitis and sometimes, syphilis, are some diseases that are transmitted through direct contact.

Transmission via fomites is also possible. These are inanimate objects that serve as a means of transmitting infections from an infected person to a healthy person. Elevator buttons, doorknobs, phones, handrails, keyboards and a host of other objects that many people share regularly are common examples of fomites.

Inhalation

Inhalation refers to the transmission of infections through aerosolized germs that are airborne until they find a susceptible person to infect.

This normally occurs when an infected person talks, coughs or sneezes. He/she releases contagious and airborne germs that are transmitted to whoever comes in contact with them. Examples of diseases that are transmitted through inhalation are measles and tuberculosis.

Sometimes, medical equipment contains aerosolized germs. Such germs are also a common feature in construction zones where dust serves as their host. Aspergillus or nontuberculous mycobacteria are transmitted through this channel.

Vector-Borne

Some infectious agents are transmitted by vectors. These organisms can transmit infections from animal to animal or human to human. Vector-borne diseases are the leading cause of mortality and morbidity in the world, although subtropical and tropical countries are most commonly hit by such diseases.

The major factors that affect vector-borne diseases are rainfall and temperature.

Some diseases that can be transmitted by vectors are:

- Lyme disease – Infected ticks spread this disease from one person to another
- Yellow fever – Aedes mosquitoes transmit the viral disease
- Chagas – The disease is transmitted through infected blood transfusions and contaminated food
- Malaria – Caused by plasmodium, a parasite transmitted via infected mosquitoes
- Lymphatic filariasis – Mosquitoes transmit filarial parasites to trigger this medical condition
- Dengue fever – Mosquitoes transmit this disease that is notorious for its lethal complications

A World Health Organization report shows that vector-borne diseases are responsible for 17% of all infectious diseases. Malaria is the most deadly disease transmitted by vectors. Dengue, another vector-borne disease, is gradually building a reputation as the fastest-growing disease in this class. Over the last five decades, the World Health Organization has reported a 30-fold increase in dengue incidences.

Ingestion

Ingestion is otherwise known as oral transmission. It occurs when a healthy person accidentally consumes contaminated water or food, leading to the ingestion of harmful organisms.

Feces, exudates, saliva or urine may contaminate an object through which the pathogenic organism may be ingested. Salmonella, campylobacter, leptospira and Escherichia coli are some common examples of diseases that are transmitted orally.

Chain of Infection

Infectious diseases can't survive in the absence of a host, an agent and an environment. Thus, they require a chain of infection that supports their existence. A deep understanding of the chain of infection may go a long way in helping medical experts and assistants to prevent and treat infectious diseases.

There are six links in the chain of infection. Each link is crucial to the chain because without it, the chain is incomplete, and transmission of such infectious diseases is impossible.

Pathogen

This may be a bacterium, virus or any other disease-causing organism.

Reservoir

The reservoir refers to the environment that assures the pathogen's survival. This may be an animal, a human or an environment. Humans may transmit an infection to each other through numerous means, as mentioned above.

Animal reservoirs are animals that transmit infections. Cows, sheep, rodents, rabbits, dogs, bats, pigs and birds are some common examples of animal reservoirs. They transmit several diseases that include brucellosis, anthrax, monkeypox, tularemia and rabies, among others.

Soil, plants and water are examples of environmental reservoirs. They serve as infectious agents for some diseases such as legionnaires and legionella pneumophila.

Portal of Exit

Portal of exit refers to the channel through which a transmission agent leaves the host's body. The location of the pathogen more often than not corresponds to the portal of exit.

For instance, mycobacterium tuberculosis affects the respiratory tract, and that serves as its portal of exit as well. The same rule applies to other infectious diseases.

Means of Transmission

The means of transmission refers to the channel through which an infection is transmitted from its natural reservoir to a host.

Portal of Entry

The portal of entry refers to the means through which the pathogen enters its host. This may be through inhalation, penetration or ingestion. It may also be through the mucous membranes as seen in syphilis, or through the skin, using hookworm as a typical example, or through the blood. HIV and hepatitis B are two examples of diseases that are transmitted through the blood.

The depth of penetration is a crucial factor in determining the severity of an infection.

New Host

The host is the final link in the infection chain. Several factors determine a host's susceptibility. These are constitutional factors, genetic factors and some specific immunity factors.

For instance, a host's resistance to infection may be increased or decreased by individual genetics. Someone with sickle cell traits is more susceptible to infections and has lower immunity to infection than others.

Infection Control

The following practices will ensure that you play your part in controlling infections while discharging your health-care responsibilities:

Maintain Hand Hygiene

As a medical assistant, you come in direct contact with patients with all forms of ailments regularly. You may be exposed to their fluids and blood on some occasions. That is aside from microscopic disease-causing organisms.

An effective preventive measure against infection transmission is proper hand hygiene. You can always decontaminate your hands with alcohol gel to kill germs. Handwashing with antibacterial soap and water is another effective option.

You should always wash your hands under the following conditions:

- When you touch mucous membranes

- When you come in contact with bodily fluids
- When you touch contaminated items, irrespective of whether you wear gloves or not
- When moving from a contaminated site to a clean site
- After touching medical equipment or other objects
- After using the restroom
- Before and after eating
- After sneezing or coughing into a tissue

Use Appropriate Personal Protective Equipment

You must always wear appropriate personal protective equipment. The equipment includes some protective items such as masks, gloves, respirators, gowns and eyewear.

With complete protective gear, you will create barriers that protect your mucous membranes, skin, respiratory tract and clothing from deadly infectious agents.

The specific equipment you use depends on what you are exposed to. Gloves are ideal when touching bodily fluids, blood, contaminated items and mucous membranes. Goggles and a surgical mask are necessary if blood or bodily fluids may splash your mouth, eyes or nose.

If there are high chances that your clothing or skin may be exposed to bodily fluids or blood, wear a protective gown.

Once you are done using the PPE, remove it immediately. Wash your hands with either soap or alcohol gel.

Cleaning and Disinfection

A medical facility is open to the public. Hence, huge human traffic, mostly patients, makes it a hub for fomites. Contaminated objects and surfaces abound. Toilets, doorknobs and sinks are typical examples of fomites in medical facilities. These are aside from the common waiting areas and client-care areas that can harbor and spread infections.

Cleaning and disinfection of such areas and fomites should be done regularly. For effective cleaning, use EPA-registered disinfectants only. They contain manufacturers' instructions with information on the amount of the disinfectant to use and the dilution ratio.

Note that organic matter and dirt affect the effectiveness of most disinfectants. Thus, it is imperative that you clean walls and floors before disinfecting them.

Waste Disposal

Waste should be properly disposed of to prevent it from serving as a breeding ground for germs.

Dispose of sharp objects in leak-proof and puncture-resistant containers. Use a red container or one correctly marked for that purpose. Using a biohazard symbol on the container is also recommended.

Discard bloodstained disposable items in biohazard bags. Such bags shouldn't be easily breakable or punctured. Ensure that you use a leak-proof bag with the appropriate biohazard symbol for easy identification.

Disposable rags, used PPE and cloths are some items you can dispose of in a biohazard bag.

Chapter Nine: Patient Intake and Documentation of Care

Your job description as a medical assistant may include opening a medical record for new patients. When documenting the medical record of a new patient, you need to gather some important data.

Type of Data in a Medical Record

The type of data needed in a medical record is classified into:

Subjective Data

Subjective data refers to the information provided by patients about themselves and their ailment. A knowledgeable companion such as a friend, spouse or other informed family member may also provide the information.

With this data, you can deduce how the patient feels, the ailment's symptoms and the person's concerns. In this category are the patient's personal data that includes:

Major Complaint: This is the first piece of information you need from the patient. What is the current medical problem the patient is seeking help for? What are the symptoms? Headache? Frequent urination at night? Excessive sweating?

Present Ailment: What ailment are the major complaints symptoms of? An interactive session with the patient will reveal the present ailment the patient is struggling with.

Family Medical History: The patient's family medical history should also be documented. It enables you to know whether there are any hereditary ailments to deal with.

Past Medical History: Aside from the patient's family medical history, past medical history should also be taken into consideration. What ailments has the patient been treated for in the past?

Social History: While the patient's medical history is very important, don't forget social history as well. For instance, smokers are more liable to some types of cancers. Excessive alcohol consumers may be prone to some other ailments as well. Thus, you must gather information about the patient's social history and document that carefully.

Occupation: Don't ignore the patient's occupation. This information may give you a clue as to what you are dealing with. For instance, it is not uncommon for people whose job exposes them to carcinogenic substances to suffer from one form of cancer or the other. People working in the construction industry may suffer from specific ailments as well.

The following are some examples of subjective data a patient may provide:

- Dizziness
- Pain
- Coughing
- Shortness of breath
- Exhaustion
- Vomiting
- Itching

Objective Data

Objective data refers to the physical data that you can personally observe and see. Contrary to the information provided by the patient, you use your senses to identify objective data.

You can't argue objective data because it is identified through different means that include tests, vitals and physical examinations.

Heart rate, weight, blood pressure, height, general appearance and body temperature are examples of objective data.

Generally, during the initial patient assessment, these are your responsibilities:

- Assessing the patient and collecting vital signs such as pulse, blood pressure, temperature and breathing rate
- Performing a physical examination on the patient
- Obtaining the patient's medical, employment and social history
- Measuring weight and height as part of the physical exam. You should also look for irregularities or deformities on the individual's body
- Recording your findings and presenting the results to the physician attending to the patient

Treatment Compliance

Treatment compliance refers to the degree to which a patient is willing to abide by medical directives, attend appointments, follow medical regimens and engage in preventive care as recommended by the patient's health-care provider.

Not every patient follows medical advice carefully. Some stop taking their medications, skip appointments or generally engage in activities that will hamper their recuperation.

Failure to follow medical directives completely may have dire consequences for a patient. Aside from hampering recovery, it may complicate a person's medical condition as well. This underscores the importance of ensuring strict compliance by patients.

Here are some helpful tips you can use to encourage more patient compliance:

Support the Patient: Rather than getting angry and scolding the patient, support the patient in whatever way you can. Some words of encouragement, practical tips and other efforts may yield a more positive result.

Public Service Campaigns: Public service campaigns can also help increase adherence to medication and general medical advice. The United States has hundreds of sponsors and partners for such campaigns, and they are a powerful tool to connect with patients and pass along the crucial message of the importance of treatment adherence.

Highlight the Importance of Compliance: Some patients may discontinue their medical treatment due to a lack of proper information about the consequences of their actions. Thus, take the time to educate patients of the need to see their treatment through and keep appointments. When you show them the huge health benefits of such action, they will be more willing to complete their treatment and do whatever is required of them.

Set Constant Reminders: Some patients are forgetful. Sometimes, it may be a symptom of a medical condition or may be triggered by some other factors. Some patients need a constant reminder to follow a medical regimen.

You may send text message reminders when necessary. This is a cost-effective and highly effective strategy that will encourage your patients to practice medication adherence. According to some analyses, such reminders may improve adherence rates by 17.8%.

Follow-Up Calls: Another effective approach is follow-up calls. While some younger patients may not appreciate this, older patients understand the rationale behind the call. When you reach out to them by phone, answer their questions, discuss treatment regimen and remind them about why complying with medical instructions and treatment is beneficial to them, there are increased chances that patients will take their treatment more seriously.

Simplify the Regimen: Some patients may find medication adherence challenging if the treatment regimen is too complex. Rather than use medical terms that may be too difficult for such individuals to understand, use common words and expressions to explain the regimen. You can also encourage patients to repeat the instructions back to you to ensure that they understand.

Educate Your Patients: It is your responsibility to teach your patients why and how they should follow a prescribed medical regimen. If there are terms or conditions they don't understand, take the time to explain. You can use illustrations, teaching aids, etc. Your patients will be more willing to take their treatments seriously if they understand their conditions and treatments better.

Factors Affecting Treatment Compliance

Patient's lackadaisical attitude towards treatment can be traced to an array of factors including:

- Complexity of the treatment
- Lack of understanding
- Medication cost
- Medication side effects
- Poor provider-patient relationship
- Cognitive impairment
- Psychological problems
- Treatment of asymptomatic disease
- Barriers to medications and care
- Inadequate follow-up

Importance of Treatment Compliance

Treatment compliance should be enforced within the medical industry. There are several reasons why you must ensure that your patients take their treatment seriously and take their medications as prescribed.

Improved Health

Medications and other medical treatments serve a purpose: to help the patient recuperate. This objective will be defeated if a patient doesn't follow medical instructions.

Cost-Effective

Treatment compliance is also cost-effective. You can imagine the cost of being readmitted to a hospital if the patient suffers a relapse. The initial treatment cost and the cost of a relapse can take a toll on the patient. This can be avoided with strict adherence to established treatment procedures.

Treatment compliance can go a long way in improving a patient's health. While some patients are apathetic towards complying with medical instructions, you can encourage them to see the reasons why taking such instructions seriously is beneficial for them.

Vital Signs Equipment

As previously mentioned, taking a patient's vital signs in preparation for an examination or a procedure is a part of your job.

The following four vital signs are the most basic functions of the body:

Blood Pressure: Blood pressure refers to the pressure in the arteries. Blood pressure is produced through the contraction of the heart muscle. When measuring blood pressure, two major components are measured. These are the systolic pressure and diastolic pressure. This refers to the measurement taken after the contraction of the heart and before the contraction, respectively. The higher figure represents the systolic pressure, while the lower figure represents the diastolic pressure.

Blood pressure is measured with a sphygmomanometer. A normal blood pressure reads below 120/80.

Temperature: Body temperature is the degree of hotness or coldness of a body. Factors such as food consumption, gender, time of day and recent activity determine a person's body temperature. However, normal body temperature ranges between 36.5°C and 37.2°C (between 97.8°F and 99°F).

Body temperature can be measured with a thermometer.

Respiratory Rate: The respiration rate of an individual is the number of breaths taken per minute. It is conventionally measured by counting the number of times the chest of a person at rest rises. Factors that may increase respiration rates include illness, fever and a host of other medical problems. A healthy adult has a normal respiration range between 12 and 16 breaths each minute.

A respirometer is used to measure respiration rate. It measures the rate at which carbon dioxide or/and oxygen is exchanged.

Pulse Rate: The pulse rate refers to the number of times a heart beats per minute. You can measure the pulse rate of a patient with a stethoscope.

A healthy adult's pulse rate lies between 60 and 100 beats per minute. Some factors that determine an individual's pulse rate are illness, emotions and exercise.

Patient Preparation and Provider Assistance

As an assistant to the physician, you perform the following duties when preparing a patient for any medical examination or procedure:

- You must first prepare the room. This involves ensuring that all the necessary instruments and equipment are available. They must all have been sanitized and disinfected. Don't forget to keep the examination room well lit, clean, at a comfortable temperature and well ventilated. Once you are done with the room preparation, move to the next stage: patient preparation.
- In preparation for the physical examination, ask the patient to disrobe if necessary. Provide an examination gown to put on. Drape the patient's legs if he/she is wearing a gown. Put the patient's chart outside the door of the examination room. Notify the physician of the patient's readiness to undergo the examination.

Chapter Ten: Nutrition

Nutrition is crucial to healthy living. The medical field always emphasizes the importance of a balanced diet, an important part of nutrition.

The CMA exam will test your knowledge of food nutrients, dietary supplements, special dietary needs and eating disorders. Let's take a comprehensive look at each of these aspects of nutrition.

Food Nutrients

Food is classified into six classes, with nutritional value as the major yardstick for the classification. These classes are:

Carbohydrates

Carbohydrates are a class of food whose molecules consist of oxygen, carbon and hydrogen atoms. They are a member of the triune classes of food collectively known as macronutrients, alongside protein and fat.

Dietary carbohydrates are divided into three categories:

Starches: Starches are long-chain glucose molecules. The digestive system breaks them down into glucose.

Sugars: These are short-chain carbohydrates. Some examples are fructose, sucrose, glucose and galactose.

Fiber: Humans can't digest fiber. Nevertheless, the digestive system contains some bacteria that can use some of the fiber.

Carbohydrates are found in foods such as vegetables, fibers, grains, starches, fruits, fibers and some dairy products.

Healthy carbohydrates can be found in nuts, vegetables, seeds, tubers, legumes, whole fruits and whole grains. So-called "bad carbs" should be consumed in smaller quantities. These include white bread, sugary drinks, pastries, ice cream, fruit juices and snacks like potato chips or fries.

Protein

Protein provides the building blocks needed by the body. Muscles, bone, cells, hair and skin all contain protein.

Protein makes up about 16% of the total body weight of an average person. Unsurprisingly, it is needed by the body for health, growth and maintenance.

The human body contains about 10,000 different proteins, each playing different roles in the body.

Some foods that are rich in protein are fish, meat and eggs. Soy, beans, some grains and nuts also contain a significant amount of protein.

Protein is a product of amino acids, otherwise known as the body's building blocks. Although the human body doesn't store amino acids, it makes them by modifying other amino acids or creating them from scratch.

Humans get nine amino acids from protein: isoleucine, histidine, lysine, threonine, leucine, tryptophan, methionine, valine and phenylalanine.

An adult needs a minimum of 0.8 grams of protein per kilogram of the individual's body weight or seven grams of protein for every 20 pounds of an adult's body weight, according to the National Academy of Medicine.

Fats

Fats were previously considered unhealthy. However, recent research has shown that a healthy diet is incomplete without healthy fats. While it is true that fat contains a high calorie content, the human body needs these calories as a source of energy.

The World Health Organization recommends limiting fats to fewer than 30% of one's daily calories.

Healthy fats help keep blood sugar under control. They also reduce the risk of type 2 diabetes and heart disease and have a positive impact on brain function.

Other important benefits of healthy fats include lowering the risk of cancer, arthritis and Alzheimer's disease, as well as being powerful anti-inflammatories.

Fats are classified into:

Saturated Fats

Saturated fats are "saturated" with hydrogen atoms. Their chemical structure gives them a solid texture at room temperature.

Some sources of saturated fats are:

- Some plant oils such as coconut oil or palm kernel
- Poultry, beef, pork and some animal meats

- Processed meats such as hot dogs, bologna, bacon and sausages
- Dairy products such as butter, cheese and milk
- Some pre-packaged snacks such as cookies, crackers, pastries and chips

The impact of saturated fats on your health depends on the source of the fat. According to a study, dairy products reduce the risk of cardiovascular disease. On the other hand, processed meats increase the risk.

Unsaturated Fats

Unsaturated fats are liquid at room temperature. Thus, they are different from their saturated counterparts.

Unsaturated fats are classified into polyunsaturated and monounsaturated fats. They contain one double bond and two or more double bonds respectively.

Examples of monounsaturated fats are olive oil and canola oil. Others are avocados, most seeds, peanut oil and most nuts.

Examples of polyunsaturated fats are sunflower, safflower oil and corn oil. Others are sunflower seeds, oysters and fatty fish such as tuna sardines, mackerel, salmon, herring and trout.

Vitamins

Vitamins are substances that the human body needs for proper development and growth. They are present in food and are essential for metabolism. Vitamin deficiencies can lead to some serious health conditions.

The human body contains 13 vitamins that include vitamin A, B, C, D, E, K and others.

Humans can get most of these types of vitamins from the food they consume, while sunlight is a good source of vitamin D.

Vitamins are classified into:

Fat-Soluble Vitamins

Fat-soluble vitamins are stored in the body's fatty tissues and liver. Due to their nature, the body can store them for days, and when necessary, for months.

Water-Soluble Vitamins

Unlike fat-soluble vitamins, water-soluble vitamins don't stay for long in the body because the body can't store them. As a result, they are passed from the body through urine. Thus, the body needs to replace them more frequently than fat-soluble vitamins.

The following are good sources of water-soluble vitamins:

- Vitamin C
- Vitamin B1 (thiamine)
- Vitamin B12
- Vitamin B6
- Vitamin B2 (riboflavin)
- Vitamin B9 (folic acid)
- Vitamin B3 (niacin)

Some good sources of vitamins are whole grains, brown rice, oranges, liver, potatoes, broccoli, spinach, yeast and sunflower seeds.

Beriberi, scurvy, pellagra and rickets are some of the medical conditions that are caused by vitamin deficiencies. Mouth ulcers, bleeding gums, poor night vision, scaly patches, hair loss and dandruff are other ailments related to vitamin deficiencies.

Minerals

Minerals serve several roles in the body. Some of their responsibilities include keeping the muscles, bones, brain and heart in peak condition. The body can't make hormones and enzymes without these essential elements.

Minerals are classified into:

Trace Minerals

Trace minerals are minerals that the human body needs in small quantities. Examples of trace minerals are manganese, iodine, iron, cobalt, zinc, selenium and fluoride.

Macro-minerals

Macro-minerals are essential minerals that the body needs in large quantities. They include potassium, calcium, chloride, magnesium, sodium and phosphorus.

Minerals perform the following functions in the body:

- Build strong bones
- Control bodily fluids, both outside and inside cells
- Convert food into energy

Water

Water is arguably the most important nutrient the human body needs. Dehydration may cause impaired physical functioning, headaches and may hamper mental ability. Severe dehydration can also lead to death.

Water serves the following purposes:

- It transports nutrients
- It removes toxins
- It lubricates body organs
- It prevents dehydration
- It prevents constipation
- It helps the body to absorb shock

Special Dietary Needs

Special dietary needs refer to specific types of foods that people with some medical conditions require for various reasons. These reasons include:

Weight Control

The following foods are recommended for weight loss:

Leafy Greens: Leafy greens such as spinach, Swiss chard and kale are low in carbohydrates and calories, making them perfect for weight loss. They are also rich in fiber. Leafy greens also contain antioxidants, vitamins and some minerals that aid fat burning.

Beans and Legumes: Some legumes and beans are great for weight loss. They are high in fiber and protein, two nutrients that support satiety. Black beans, lentils and kidney beans are examples of foods in this group.

Whole Grains: Whole grains (as opposed to refined grains) are loaded with protein and fiber. Some whole grains, such as oats, also possess soluble fiber that improves metabolic health and ensures satiety.

Fruits: It can be argued that fruits contain natural sugar. However, unlike artificial sugar, their low energy density makes them healthy. They also contain fiber that regulates the rate at which sugar is released into the bloodstream. Hence, fruits are healthy.

Hypertension

Hypertension is otherwise known as high blood pressure. This medical condition can trigger a stroke if not treated immediately.

Hypertensive people can manage their condition by consuming foods that are low in cholesterol, saturated fat, added sugars and salt. They should also eat foods that are rich in protein, nutrients and fiber.

Excessive sodium consumption can increase the body's fluid retention, leading to increased blood pressure.

The foods listed below are recommended for hypertensive people:

- Fruit
- Fish
- Whole grains
- Nuts
- Poultry
- Low-fat or fat-free products

Hypertensive individuals should avoid:

- Added sugars
- Red meats, including lean red meats
- Sugar-containing drinks
- Sweets

Cancer

Cancer patients should increase their protein consumption to enable the body to repair the damaging side effects that may arise from treating the ailment. Cancer patients are prone to malnutrition, thanks to their loss of appetite, taste and smell occasioned by the medical condition or its treatment.

Good high-protein foods for cancer patients to consume include eggs, lean meat, cheese, chicken, nuts, yogurt, beans and fish.

Cancer patients should also ensure they stay well hydrated.

Lactose Intolerance or Sensitivity

Lactose is a type of sugar that is commonly found in animal milk. The lactase enzyme breaks lactose down and digests it.

However, someone who is lactase intolerant doesn't have enough lactase and may develop symptoms such as vomiting, bloating, stomach cramps and diarrhea.

Lactose intolerant individuals shouldn't consume canned tuna, sauces, gravy, sweeteners and beer.

Lactose-free products are derived from cow's milk. The right amount of enzyme is added to neutralize the lactose effect on consumers.

Potato chips and soy products such as milk proteins and cheese are also good for such individuals.

Eating Disorders

Eating disorders are medical conditions that impact people's eating behaviors and adversely affect their emotions, health and ability to function properly.

Eating disorders are considered a mental health condition that can only be solved by psychological and medical experts. An estimated 30 million Americans struggle with an eating disorder.

Eating disorders are usually triggered by an unusual obsession with one's body weight, food or body shape.

There are six different types of eating disorders. They are:

Anorexia Nervosa

Anorexia nervosa is more common in women than men and typically develops during young adulthood or adolescence. People with the medical condition view themselves as always overweight, although that may be quite far from the truth. In some cases, anorexia nervosa patients are actually underweight. As a result of their misconception about their weight, they avoid foods they believe contribute to their weight and limit their caloric consumption.

Some common symptoms of this health condition are:

- Restricted eating patterns
- Considerably underweight
- Irrational fear of gaining any weight

Binge-Eating

This is one of the leading eating disorders in the United States. Most binge eaters are young adults and adolescents. Sometimes, though, older people may also develop this medical condition.

Binge eaters compulsively consume large amounts of food within a short period of time.

Some common symptoms of binge-eating disorders are:

- Inability to control themselves while binge-eating
- Feeling disgust, shame or guilt when eating
- Eating until they are uncomfortably full, regardless of whether they are actually hungry or not

Rumination Disorders

Rumination disorder refers to an eating disorder in which the victim regurgitates previously chewed food, re-chews the food, re-swallows it or spits it out.

Patients engage in this practice within half or an hour of having a meal. This eating disorder can develop at any stage of life: childhood, infancy or adulthood. While infants get over this condition naturally, adults and children require professional assistance.

Other eating disorders include restrictive/avoidant food intake disorder, pica and bulimia nervosa. Eating disorders can be destructive if not properly managed.

Chapter Eleven: Specimen Collection

Specimen collection refers to the process through which medical practitioners obtain fluids or tissues for laboratory analysis or patient testing.

Without specimen collection and analysis, diagnosis may be impossible, and treating a patient without diagnosis of their medical condition is unethical.

Stool, urine and sputum are some specimens that are frequently collected for analysis. A venipuncture can also be performed on a patient to collect a blood sample.

Importance of Specimen Collection

Proper specimen collection has the following benefits for medical providers:

- It makes it easier to provide quality care
- It makes it easier to diagnose and treat health problems
- It saves time and money as it guarantees more efficient treatment
- It reduces the risk of exposure to pathogens and/or accidental injury

For the patient, the benefits of proper specimen collection include:

- Accurate, swift diagnosis and treatment
- It prevents unnecessary testing and therefore saves time and money

Types of Specimens

Different types of specimens are used for laboratory analyses. These are:

Blood Specimen

Blood is one of the most commonly collected specimens due to its use for a wide range of diagnoses.

Some common methods for collecting blood specimens are:

Venipuncture

A venipuncture is a process through which blood is collected from a vein for laboratory testing.

There are two major parts of the body where blood specimens can be taken. These are the veins located inside of the elbow or those on top of the hand.

Only experienced, trained health workers are allowed to use this method to collect blood specimens. This is to prevent some of the risks common to the procedure, such as fainting, infection, blood accumulation under the skin (hematoma), feeling lightheaded and excessive bleeding.

Venipuncture Equipment

Some special equipment is needed to perform a venipuncture. This includes:

- Gauze
- Needles
- Gloves
- Collection tubes or evacuated tubes
- Bandages
- Wipes or swabs
- Disposal unit
- Tourniquet
- Tube additives

Venipuncture Procedure

The venipuncture procedure is as follows:

Gather the Equipment: Collect all the necessary equipment prior to beginning the procedure.

Prep the Patient: After collecting the equipment, prepare the patient for the procedure. Start off by introducing yourself to make the patient feel comfortable. Ask for the patient's name as well. Check if the patient's name matches the name on the laboratory form. Does the patient have any allergies? Also, find out if the patient has ever had complications while having blood drawn.

Locate the Vein: Locate the vein for specimen collection by asking the patient to extend his/her hand. Look for the most clearly visible vein before applying the tourniquet. Apply the tourniquet three to four inches above the site you will use for the venipuncture.

Sanitize your Hands: Wash your hands with soap and water and clean them with a single-use towel. Alternatively, clean your hands with an alcohol wipe.
Put on your gloves once you have thoroughly washed your hands.

Disinfect the Venipuncture Site: Do this before the procedure as a preventive measure against contamination. For the cleaning, use a 70% alcohol swab. Start from the center of the site and clean outwards. The cleaning should cover between two and four centimeters.

After cleaning, allow the disinfected area to dry before the procedure. The risk of contamination is thereby reduced. Don't touch the site after cleaning to prevent contamination. If you accidentally touch it, repeat the disinfecting process.

An alternative disinfectant sometimes used is povidone iodine. However, it gives false lab test results. So, avoid using iodine and follow the other disinfection procedures described here.

Draw the Blood: Put your thumb below the venipuncture site while the patient forms a fist with his/her hand. With the needle held at a 30-degree angle, puncture the vein as quickly as possible. Release the tourniquet after collecting the blood. Then, remove the needle slowly. Use a cotton ball or clean gauze to apply pressure to the site.

For multiple blood collection, use evacuated tubes with a tube holder and a needle to enable you to fill the tubes directly. Alternatively, use a winged needle set or a syringe for the same purpose. Before filling the tube, place it into a rack.

Discard Used Equipment: Complete the procedure by discarding used equipment into a Sharps container or any other puncture-resistant container. Use a general waste container for disposing of items with no blood on them.

Prepare the Blood Sample: Put the collected samples into a leak-proof and sealed bag in preparation for transportation. If you collected multiple samples, put the tubes in a rack for transportation to avoid cross-contamination and breakage.

Dermal Puncture

Another effective blood-collecting technique for laboratory analysis is a dermal puncture. This procedure is used for collecting blood from capillaries. Since capillaries are between veins and arteries, the blood collected through this technique is a mixture of blood from the arteries and veins.

This technique requires less precision than the venipuncture technique. Thus, it is the preferred blood-taking technique of choice for infants.

The technique also requires less blood. When a large quantity of blood is needed for some laboratory tests, a dermal puncture is not an appropriate collection technique.

A dermal puncture is more time-consuming than the venipuncture process. This may have a huge impact on the outcome of whatever test is done with the collected specimen.

For instance, the delay may result in a medical condition such as hemolysis or blood clotting. The blood or fluid being collected may also be contaminated. That may lead to inaccurate test results.

Note also that a dermal puncture is not ideal for patients with poor peripheral circulation or dehydrated patients.

Urine Specimen

Aside from blood, urine collection is another common diagnostic technique. The timing, the collection technique and handling are some factors that determine the clinical information a medical team can obtain from a urine specimen.

Morning Specimen

As the name implies, this urine specimen is taken in the morning. The collected urine sample is usually more concentrated, thanks to the long duration of urine in the bladder over the night. Thus, the urine contains a higher level of analytes and cellular elements, which can enhance the accuracy of tests.

This specimen must be collected as soon as the patient wakes up. It is also known as an eight-hour specimen because the specimen can be collected within a time frame of eight hours.

Random Specimen

Random specimen refers to a urine specimen that can be taken at any time of the day. Due to the ease of taking the specimen, it remains the most popular form of specimen used for analysis. It is largely used for microscopic analysis and urinalysis. However, there is a shortcoming: the results sometimes give false and misleading information about a patient's health, especially if the specimen is overdiluted.

Catheter Collection Specimen

This is the most effective urine collection technique for patients who can't urinate without medical assistance or who are bedridden. To collect the urine specimen with this method, a Foley catheter is inserted through the urethra into the bladder. Alternatively, the specimen may be collected into an evacuated tube from a Foley. A syringe may also be used for transferring the specimen into a cup or a tube.

Midstream Clean-Catch

This technique guarantees a higher level of accuracy than some of the other alternatives. Before the specimen-taking process, the patient must use a castile soap towelette to cleanse the urethral area. Then, the first portion of the urine is voided as a preventive measure against obtaining contaminated urine.

Then, the medical worker will collect the urine mainstream into a clean container, and the excess will be flushed down the toilet. There are no specific times of the day for this collection technique.

Timed 24-Hour Collection

This collection technique requires attention to detail. To start with, the urine in the bladder should be voided and discarded. Then, the urine collection begins with the next urination, and batches of urine are collected over the next 24 hours. The urine is collected in a large collection bottle and preserved with the addition of a preservative to prevent urinary components from breakdown. Alternatively, the collected urine should be refrigerated.

You should note that none of the urine collected within the time frame should be discarded. Otherwise, you will be working with an incomplete urine sample. That may adversely affect the result of the analysis.

Sputum Specimen

People with lung-related medical conditions or a respiratory tract infection produce sputum. The excessive production of the thick substance can trigger health problems that include coughing and breathing difficulties. Sputum collection may be done to help diagnose the problem.

The following medical conditions may require a sputum test:

- Breathing difficulties
- Fatigue
- Muscle ache
- Cough
- Confusion
- Chills
- Chest pain

The diagnosis resulting from the sputum specimen may reveal underlying conditions such as:

- Pneumonia
- Cystic fibrosis
- Bronchitis
- Tuberculosis

- Lung abscess
- Chronic obstructive pulmonary disease

Specimen Collection Guidelines

A contaminated specimen won't give accurate results, and that may lead to a health provider making the wrong diagnosis and providing inappropriate treatment. A misdiagnosed patient's health is severely at risk.

The following guidelines can help a medical worker ensure accurate specimen collection:

- All containers for transporting specimens should be free of particles and very clean
- Break-resistant containers are better than glass for collection and transportation
- Once used, the container should be discarded and never reused
- The collection tubes or container should be properly labeled

Laboratory Quality Control

Laboratory quality control is the process by which analytical errors are detected in the lab. It supports accurate and reliable test results that enable medical health-care providers to provide patients with the best care. It also prevents delayed treatment and misdiagnosis, problems that may not only affect the patient negatively but also lead to increased treatment cost.

Quality control measures the precision of the system's measurement; its ability to produce accurate results over time under different conditions.

Some of the ways that quality control can be enforced are:

Test Protocols

Test protocols refer to a collection of test cases designed to check a specific part of a system. Each of the test cases should contain some important information, such as the purpose of the test, the criteria for acceptance and requirements that must be met before the test.

Daily Equipment Maintenance

For the outcome of an analysis to be considered good enough to be used by a physician, it must be accurate and reliable.

Thus, as a part of ensuring laboratory quality control, laboratory equipment used for specimen collection and for performing other related tasks must be in pristine condition. Using contaminated equipment for specimen collection exposes the sample to foreign bodies that may influence the result.

Reagent Storage

The storage method used for a reagent may also affect the quality of a test. When reagents are not properly stored, the reagent may not work as expected, and that can have a huge impact on the result.

Don't leave new reagents sitting on a desk for long. The datasheet contains storage instructions for the reagent. Read the instructions and store the reagent accordingly.

Specimens are collected for analysis purposes. However, to ensure that an analysis gives an accurate result, it must be properly done. Following the standard specimen collection guidelines will ensure that you correctly collect a specimen, to the benefit of both the patient and his/her health-care providers.

Chapter Twelve: Pharmacology

Pharmacology is a branch of science that deals with the study of drugs and their effects on consumers.

As a medical assistant, it is mandatory that you are aware of the classes of drugs, methods of drug storage and dosage.

Classes of Drugs

Drugs are classified into six classes with distinct effects, characteristics and side effects. These are:

Depressants

Depressants are a class of drugs that affects the central nervous system. They inhibit the system's functions and limit the user's abilities. Depressants cause symptoms such as relaxation, sleep, drowsiness, decreased inhibition, death, anesthesia and coma.

Depressants are considered the most widely used drugs around the world. Some known depressants are:

Barbiturates: Another name for barbiturates is downers. This is a central nervous system depressant whose major effects are a sense of relaxation and euphoria. Barbiturates affect the user's sleep patterns and are known for suppressing REM sleep. They are an addictive substance and can be abused.

Ethyl alcohol: Ethyl alcohol is generally known as alcohol. It is the world's most widely used psychoactive drug, next to caffeine. Although alcohol isn't an illegal substance, it is addictive and can be abused.

Benzodiazepines: Benzodiazepines are a class of psychoactive drugs used for treating insomnia and anxiety. They are ranked among the most widely used depressants in the US.

Depressants can have either short-term or long-term effects. In the short-term, they may produce the following effects:

- Fatigue
- Fever
- Depression
- Lowered blood pressure
- Addiction
- Virtual disturbances

- Inability or difficulty urinating
- Poor concentration
- Slow brain function

Other effects of depressants are:

- Chronic fatigue
- Depression
- Sexual problems
- Chronic breathing difficulties
- Sleep problems
- High body temperature
- Hallucinations
- Agitation
- Convulsions
- Delirium
- Diabetes
- High blood sugar
- Weight gain

Depressants do have some beneficial uses and are used to treat a wide range of medical conditions that include:

- Depression
- Seizures
- Social phobia
- Insomnia
- Obsessive-compulsive disorder
- Panic disorders

Stimulants

Stimulants are known for their ability to increase a consumer's energy and alertness temporarily.

Prescription stimulants are available as capsules or tablets. It is not uncommon to see them abused in different forms. Some abusers snort them, while others crush or inject them in liquid form. Amphetamines and cocaine are commonly abused stimulants.

Stimulants can have either short-term or long-term effects on users. Users can experience some short-term effects such as apathy, exhaustion and depression.

Addiction to stimulants can result in overdosing on the drug. Over a short period, high-dose usage can make the user become paranoid or hostile. Other effects include irregular heartbeat and high body temperature.

Some commonly used stimulants are pseudoephedrine and methylphenidate.

Some of the effects of stimulants include:

- Increased alertness
- Increased blood pressure
- Euphoria
- Increased heart rate
- Reduced appetite
- The desire to talk excessively

Higher doses may cause the following health problems:

- Seizures
- Tension
- Coma
- Anxiety
- Death
- Nausea
- Increased body temperature
- Tremors

Inhalants

Inhalants are a general name for substances that are inhaled to provide mind-altering or psychoactive effects on the user. The chemical vapor inhaled is absorbed into the bloodstream through the lungs. From the bloodstream, the inhalants are quickly transported to the brain and other body organs. If not controlled, inhalants can cause irreversible mental and physical damage.

While a long list of abused substances can make the list of inhalants, the term originally refers to the following substances:

Aerosol Sprays: These include hair sprays, spray paints, deodorant sprays, vegetable oil sprays and aerosol cleaning products.

Solvents: Solvents are classified into office solvents and industrial/household products. In the former class are lighter fluid, paint thinners, gasoline, dry-cleaning fluids and paint remover. Felt-tip marker fluid, glue, correction fluid and electronic contact cleaners make up the latter group.

Nitrites: This is another class of inhalant used for its psychoactive effects on consumers. Room deodorizer, video head cleaner, and leather cleaner are examples of inhaled nitrites.

Gases: Some anesthesia gases make the list of gases that are used as inhalants. These are chloroform, ether and nitrous oxide. Commercial or household gases that are used for the same purpose include propane tanks, butane lighters and whipped cream aerosols.

Some inhalants naturally affect the central nervous system and hamper brain activity.

Inhalants may cause the following short-term effects:

- Euphoria
- Distorted or slurred speech
- Lack of coordination
- Dizziness

Inhalants may also trigger these long-term problems:

- Hearing loss
- Liver damage
- Delayed behavioral development resulting from brain problems
- Kidney damage
- Brain damage resulting from insufficient oxygen flow to the brain

Hallucinogens

Hallucinogens are a group of drugs that may cause perceptual anomalies, hallucinations, and changes in the user's emotions, thoughts and consciousness.

Some hallucinogens are human-made, while mushrooms and plants are the sources of others. These substances have been used for years for healing and religious rituals. Recently, people have found other uses for these substances as they are now used for recreational and social purposes.

Some common hallucinogens are:

Mescaline: Mescaline occurs naturally in the peyote cactus. The plant's top contains a disc-shaped part where mescaline can be found. The mescaline container can be dried out and soaked in liquid or chewed for its intoxicating effect. Aside from the natural source, mescaline can also be made synthetically.

Psilocybin: Psilocybin is a natural substance housed by some hallucinogenic mushrooms that contain psilocin and psilocybin.

LSD: D-lysergic acid diethylamide is made from ergot. The man-made chemical is arguably the most powerful member of this class of drugs. It causes hallucinations.

Other common examples of hallucinogens are PCP, ayahuasca and DMT (dimethyltryptamine). Hallucinogens are otherwise known as dissociative drugs.

Cannabis

Globally, marijuana or cannabis is undoubtedly the most popular and commonly used illegal drug. This mood-altering drug is classified as a Schedule 1 controlled substance due to its huge impact on nearly every body organ.

It is made up of over 120 compounds with potentially different properties found in the leaves, flowering tops, seeds and stems of the cannabis sativa plant, otherwise known as hemp.

Marijuana can be used for treating muscle spasticity, chronic pain, nausea, anorexia and sleep disturbances. The medical form of marijuana isn't standardized by the government and isn't considered illegal throughout the United States.

Recreational marijuana may have a different effect on a user than the medical form. Its effects include a feeling of relaxation, lightheadedness, reduced blood pressure and increased appetite.

Regular cannabis use can trigger the following medical conditions:

- Selective impairment of cognitive functions
- Reduction in birth weight in pregnant women
- If used by schizophrenic patients, it can worsen the condition
- Impairment of body organs

Opioids

Opioids are a class of drug that relieve pain by acting on the nervous system. The opium poppy plant is the primary source of opioids, and the drug can have a variety of effects on the user.

Many opioids are prescribed for treating moderate pain by leveraging the drug's ability to block pain signals between the body and the brain. Opioids can also have a happy or feel-good effect on consumers. Thus, users are more likely to become addicted.

Opioids' negative side effects include constipation, slowed breathing, confusion, nausea and drowsiness.

Individuals who use opioids regularly are at risk of developing a dependence and tolerance for the drug. Hence, they may resort to using the drug at every given opportunity, as well as using higher dosages to meet their needs. This may lead to addiction over time. Overdosing on the drug can have fatal consequences.

Opioids include fentanyl, heroin, oxycodone, morphine, hydrocodone, codeine and others.

Drug Storage Methods

Medications can be damaged by several factors that include excessive exposure to light, heat and moisture. Exposure to such conditions can make drugs become toxic when ingested or destroy their potency.

Hence, the safety and potency of medications are affected by how they are stored. This underlines the importance of proper storage for all types of medications.

There are no one-size-fits-all storage methods for medications. Each medication has a storage method recommended by the manufacturer. Therefore, it is advisable that you check the recommended storage instructions and abide by them. This involves paying attention to conditions such as refrigeration, room temperature and freezing.

Storing medications at room temperature means they should be stored between 15 and 25°C. 8 to 15°C is the ideal storage temperature for medications that are meant to be stored at cool temperatures. For refrigerated medication, the ideal temperature is between 2 and 8°C. -10 to -25°C is the recommended temperature for medications that are meant to be stored at freezing temperatures.

A common storage instruction is to store medications in a cool and dry place, away from children. Obviously, this is to prevent exposure to sunlight and other elements that may affect their potency and to prevent accidental ingestion by children.

Proper medication storage has these benefits:

- Prevents deterioration, contamination and infestation
- Reduces losses or theft
- Maintains a drug's potency and quality throughout its shelf-life
- Prevents people from using ineffective or contaminated drugs that may trigger other medical conditions aside from the health problem such drugs are primarily meant to treat

Storage Environment

You must consider several factors when choosing the most appropriate storage environment for drugs. Some of these factors include:

- Sufficient lighting without direct exposure to sunlight
- Cold storage facilities, according to the storage instructions
- Cleanliness
- Humidity control

Drug Adverse Reactions

Drug adverse reactions are dangerous, unexpected reactions to a medication.

An adverse reaction is also referred to as an adverse drug reaction (ADR), adverse drug event (ADE) or adverse event.

Adverse drug reactions are classified into:

Allergic: When a patient has a history of previous exposure to a drug, an allergic drug reaction may arise. It is usually the result of the immune system's negative reaction to a specific drug the patient has previously used. Later exposure to a drug after the initial exposure may trigger an allergic reaction.

Dose-Related: This refers to the exaggeration of the therapeutic effect of the administered drug on the user. It occurs when the drug seemingly overperforms, leading to some side effects. For instance, a diabetic may develop dose-related drug reactions such as sweating, weaknesses or nausea if the administered drug reduces the person's blood sugar level below the normal level.

Idiosyncratic: While the two reactions above are common, this reaction is mostly triggered by mechanisms that are not understood. Thus, the reaction is unpredictable. Although the reaction isn't common, it can be very serious and may include jaundice, rashes, decreased white blood cell count, anemia and nerve injury leading to impaired hearing, vision or kidney damage.

Some factors that determine the severity of adverse drug reactions include:

Drug Factors: Some drug factors determine how severely someone will react to a drug. Such factors include treatment duration, administration route, dosage, drug type and bioavailability.

Hereditary Factors: Hereditary factors may also play a huge role in some people's responses to drugs. If a patient's family has a history of allergy to certain drugs, they will more likely respond negatively to such drugs too.

Certain Ailments and Diseases: Some diseases can change people's metabolism and their response to drugs. They can also have a huge impact on drug absorption and elimination, factors that can significantly increase a consumer's vulnerability to adverse drug reactions.

Age: People of different ages react differently to drugs. Young children and infants have low metabolisms and therefore have higher chances of responding negatively to drugs than adults.

Older people are also at risk of adverse drug reactions. Some underlying health problems may increase their vulnerability; a weakened liver can have reduced metabolic power over some drugs, and the kidneys' ability to eliminate drugs may be reduced as well.

Thus, elderly individuals are more likely to experience the following side effects of some drugs: depression, lightheadedness, impaired coordination, loss of appetite, confusion and depression, among others.

A severe adverse reaction to drugs may lead to these serious consequences:

- Disability
- Death
- Congenital abnormality

Physicians' Desk Reference (PDR)

The *Physicians' Desk Reference* is an annually published reference guide for physicians. The voluminous book is a list of all the licensed drugs across the United States. These drugs are approved by the Food and Drug Administration (FDA) and are published with the assistance of the pharmaceutical companies in the country.

Drug manufacturers provide the information included in the book. Thus, the book contains extensive information on approved drugs, including product or prescribing information.

In the *Physicians' Desk Reference*, you will find the following information about each of the listed drugs:

- Manufacturer
- Drug name
- Description
- Dosage and indications
- Pharmacokinetics
- Common brand names

- Adverse reactions
- DEA class, whether it is a prescription drug or not
- Supply method (injection or liquid)
- Drug interactions
- Contact information for state DEA programs
- Each state's contact information for drug and poison control centers
- Controlled substance categories

The *Physicians' Desk Reference* is divided into six color-coded sections:

Section 1: This is the manufacturer's index where you can find important information such as the manufacturer, manufacturer's address, page numbers of where you can find some additional information on the specific drug and a list of other products made by the manufacturer.

Section 2: This section contains page numbers for the drug. The generic names and brand names are used for the pagination. This section is useful when looking up unfamiliar drug names.

Section 3: This is the product category index. If you know a drug's actions but not the name, this section is useful.

Section 4: This section provides a valuable guide for product identification. The drugs can be identified by their photos, manufacturers' names and/or names listed in alphabetical order.

Section 5: This is the product information section. You can use it to find important information such as drug dosage and potential side effects.

Section 6: This is the diagnostic product information section. The information here is provided by manufacturer name, arranged alphabetically. The diagnostic guideline of each drug that isn't accompanied by official package information is available in this section.

Drug Administration Techniques

Drugs are administered in several ways. Some common drug administration techniques are:

Oral Administration: Oral drug administration can include capsules, liquids, chewable tablets or swallowed tablets. It can be argued that the oral route is the safest, most convenient and least expensive drug administration method.

Drugs administered orally move to the liver through the intestinal walls. From there, they are transported to the target site through the bloodstream.

Subcutaneous Route: This is a form of drug administration performed through injection. A needle is inserted beneath the skin. After injection, the drug moves into the capillaries or small blood vessels on its way to the bloodstream.

Intramuscular Route: This is the preferred route when there is a need to inject a patient with a large quantity of medication. The drugs are injected into the muscles below the fatty tissues and the skin. Hence, they require longer needles than the ones used for subcutaneous injections. The most common sites for intramuscular drug administration are the muscles of the thigh, the upper arms or the buttocks. The volume of blood supplied to the muscle determines the absorption rate of the injected drug.

Vaginal Route: Sometimes, drug administration is done vaginally through a tablet, solution, ring or gel. A typical example of a vaginally administered drug is estrogen. Menopausal women use this drug to treat some vaginal medical conditions such as soreness, dryness and redness.

The choice of the most appropriate way to administer a drug is dependent on three factors. These are:

- The part of the body to be treated
- The drug's formula
- How the drug works

Chapter Thirteen: First Aid

First aid treatment is fundamental knowledge expected of every medical professional.

It is usually the first form of treatment offered to someone suffering from a sudden ailment or injury. The objective is to offer the individual the necessary assistance and prevent the situation from deteriorating until the patient can receive higher-level medical care.

When offering first aid, follow these steps:

Check the Scene for Signs of Potential Danger: This may include the primary cause of the problem. This may give you a clue into the best way to handle the health problem.

Call for Medical Assistance if Necessary: While you're on the scene, you may notice things that pose a big health risk. Is there falling debris? Do you see signs of fire? If you identify anything that may endanger you and the victim, leave the scene immediately and call for medical assistance.

On the other hand, if there are no signs of danger, assess the victim's condition and do not leave him/her unless it is absolutely necessary.

Provide Care Immediately: If there are no potential signs of danger at the scene, do whatever you can to immediately assist the injured or sick person.

Some minor injuries that may be efficiently treated with first aid are:

- Cuts
- Burns
- Splinters
- Strains
- Abrasions or scrapes
- Sprains
- Stings
- Nasal congestion
- Fever
- Sore throat
- Cough

First Aid Kit

A first aid kit may contain any of the following equipment:

- Sterile eye dressings
- Safety pins
- A pair of scissors
- Different sizes of Band-Aids
- Disposable sterile gloves
- Crepe-rolled and triangular bandages
- Distilled water
- Painkillers
- Antihistamine tablets or cream
- Adhesive tape
- Small flashlight
- Antacids
- Cigarette lighter
- Oral decongestants
- Allergy medications

Emergency Identification and Response

Your ability to identify emergency situations and respond to them appropriately will also be tested during the CMA examination.

It is imperative that you understand the best way to respond to the following emergencies:

Choking

People can choke when a foreign object blocks airflow by lodging in the victim's windpipe or throat. This is usually caused by food or a foreign object.

When airflow is blocked, the brain is denied the oxygen it needs to keep functioning. Hence, first aid must be provided immediately.

Some universal signs of choking are:

- Talking difficulty
- Flushed skin that may subsequently turn bluish or pale
- Noisy or difficult breathing
- Loss of consciousness
- Lips, skin and nails turning dusky or blue

If the individual can still cough, let him/her continue coughing. Otherwise, do the following to clear the windpipe:

- Give the patient five back blows. If you are treating an adult, stand behind the person and to the side. Bend the individual at the waist and give five back blows with the heel of your hand. Target the person's shoulder blades for the blows. Kneel down behind a child to deliver the blows.
- Give the patient five abdominal thrusts as well.
- Alternate between the five thrusts and five blows until you clear the blockage.

Bleeding

Excessive bleeding, if not promptly attended to and stopped, can lead to a series of medical conditions. In extreme cases, it can result in death.

This is a step-by-step guide to stop bleeding:

- Use a clean cloth to apply direct pressure on the wound. Alternatively, use a piece of gauze or tissue until the bleeding stops.
- Don't remove the material if blood soaks through it. Rather, put more material on the wound and keep applying pressure.
- If the leg or arm is affected, raise the affected part above the heart to slow the bleeding.
- Once you are done, wash your hands thoroughly before you clean and dress the wound.
- Unless it is absolutely necessary, especially if the bleeding is so severe that direct pressure application makes no impact, don't apply a tourniquet.

Sometimes, calling a doctor may be the best assistance you can render. It is the best solution if there is:

- A deep wound
- A wound with gaping or jagged edges
- Numbness around the wound
- A wound caused by human or animal bite
- Signs of infection such as thick discharge, tenderness or redness
- Fever
- Debris or dirt in the wound
- Internal bleeding

Cold Exposure

Intense cold can have a damaging effect on people's health. It can lead to a huge drop in the patient's overall temperature, a condition medically known as hypothermia. It can also cause frostbite when the body's cells freeze. Either of these medical conditions can lead to death.

When providing first aid to someone suffering from cold exposure, do the following:

- Do whatever you can to raise the individual's body temperature. For frostbite, use a loose and soft cloth to wrap the area and then call for immediate medical attention. You may wrap a victim of hypothermia in dry blankets or a sleeping bag after removing any wet clothing.
- Give a conscious patient warm liquid such as hot soup or tea. Don't give alcohol-containing beverages. They can worsen the condition, especially hypothermia.
- If the person isn't coughing, breathing or moving, perform CPR.

For hypothermia:

- Never heat the person with a hot bath or a heating lamp. Heating should be done gradually.
- Do not warm a patient's legs and arms. Do not massage them either. Both of these cause damage to the lungs and heart.
- Don't offer the person cigarettes and alcohol as these can interfere with the warming process or cause more damage. Tobacco prevents circulation, while alcohol prevents the warming process.

Poisoning

Poisoning is death or injury caused by inhaling, injecting, swallowing or touching chemicals, harmful drugs, gases or venom.

The most effective first aid depends largely on the type of poisoning you are dealing with.

- For swallowed poison, remove whatever is left in the person's mouth. If a chemical or household cleaner is the poison, read and follow the instructions on the container's label for a guide on dealing with accidental poisoning.
- If the poison is in the eye, flush the eye with lukewarm water gently for about 15 minutes.
- For inhaled poison, quickly take the person out into the fresh air.
- If the person doesn't show any signs of life, start CPR immediately.
- If the poisoning leads to vomiting, turn the person to the side as a preventive measure against choking.
- If you call for an ambulance, gather the packages, pill bottles or containers that can give you some clue to the poison. The medical team may need that information when treating the victim.

A note of warning: Don't give the patient anything such as syrup of ipecac to induce vomiting. While this practice was endorsed some years back, experts now warn that inducing vomiting has proven to be ineffective and most often causes more harm.

Asthma Attack

Asthma is a chronic disease characterized by the inflammation and swelling of the bronchial tubes' lining. It usually causes difficulty in breathing.

When assisting asthmatic patients, consider the following:

- Does the person have an asthma plan? If he/she does, follow the plan. It should provide you with details about the asthma medication the individual uses and other useful information.
- Sit the person up.
- Remove tight clothing, if any. Or, loosen tight clothing around the neck.
- Assist the person in administering medication or in using their inhaler. If someone doesn't own an inhaler, don't borrow from anyone. You may find one in the first aid kit. If so, use it.
- Call for medical help as soon as possible.

Note the following:

- If wheezing stops, it is wrong to assume the condition is improving.
- Drowsiness shouldn't be mistaken for improvement. It can also mean the situation is worsening.

Insect Bite

Nearly everyone has been stung or bitten by an insect at some point.

Some symptoms of an insect bite are:

- Swelling
- Itching
- Redness
- Pain
- Breathing difficulty
- Vomiting
- Abdominal cramps
- Swelling of the lips, face or throat
- Shock

You can assist someone who has been bitten or stung with these simple medical procedures:

- Remove the embedded stinger or tick by scraping the surface gently using a flat-edged object. Don't use tweezers for the removal as that tends to release more venom as you squeeze the area affected by the sting.
- Use soap and water to wash the affected area.
- Wrap an ice pack or cold compress in a cloth and place on the area to reduce the swelling and pain. Ten minutes should suffice.
- To relieve the pain and itching, apply a paste of water and baking soda to the area. Alternatively, you can use calamine lotion.

If the patient shows a severe allergic reaction such as dizziness, wheezing or a fast heart rate, then use the following emergency treatment:

- Call 911
- If you have an epinephrine auto-injector on you, use it according to the directions
- Encourage the victim to stay calm and still.
- Elevate the victim's legs to ease any pain
- Turn the victim to the side if he/she starts vomiting
- Start CPR if the person stops breathing or remains unconscious

The following medications are effective for relieving the symptoms of insect stings or bites:

- Itching can be treated with hydrocortisone cream, crotamiton lotion or cream, antihistamine tablets or hydrocortisone ointment
- Ibuprofen and paracetamol are effective for treating discomfort or pain resulting from the sting or bite
- Antihistamine tablets are also great for reducing swelling

Note: Don't give the patient any food or drink. Don't use a tourniquet on the affected area.

Seizures

Seizures are signs of a medical condition known as epilepsy. Epilepsy is caused by a wide range of factors such as illness, brain diseases, injury or genetics.

Seizures have a wide range of symptoms that include:

- Lip smacking
- Loss of sensation

- Clouded awareness
- Convulsions
- Fidgeting
- Muscle contractions
- Confusion

Seizures usually last between 30 seconds and two minutes.

When providing assistance to someone having a seizure, do the following:

- Loosen anything that may make breathing difficult. This may include ties, clothing and jewelry
- Don't restrain the victim
- Don't put anything in the person's mouth
- Don't force the mouth open
- Don't hold the tongue
- If there are objects that can injure the person in the vicinity, remove them
- Support the person's head with something soft and flat
- Lay the victim on his/her side after the seizure to make breathing easier
- Constantly reassure the person
- Do not leave the person's side immediately after the seizure ends

Cardiac Arrest

Cardiac arrest is a sudden loss of breathing, heart function and consciousness. This medical condition is usually triggered when the heart experiences a sudden electrical disturbance. Cardiac arrest is a deadly medical condition that should be attended to with urgency.

- If you notice no sign of life in the victim, start CPR immediately.
- To keep the patient alive, perform a CPR count of between 100 and 120 pushes per minute in the center of the patient's chest. This gives the chest enough room to return to its normal position before the next push.
- If an automated external defibrillator is available, use it.
- Continue CPR until the patient recovers or medical help arrives.

Note that cardiac arrest is not synonymous with a heart attack. The former is a medical condition that arises when the heart muscle is deprived of blood due to blockage of blood flow to the muscle.

Accidents

Your response to an accident depends on the type of accident it is. Generally, if someone is injured during an accident, it is advisable to provide first aid on the spot. This may require that you perform CPR on the patient in some severe cases, after calling for help.

Joint Sprains/Dislocation

Sprains are ligament injuries. They occur when the ligament's fibers are partially or completely torn. Someone may experience a knee, wrist, ankle or thumb sprain, although ankle sprains are most common.

Some common signs and symptoms of sprains are:

- Pain in the muscle or joint
- Bruising and swelling in the affected areas
- Trouble or difficulty moving the affected areas
- Redness and warmth in the injured area

For the first 48 hours after the incidence, use RICE to assist the victim:

- **R**est: Have the victim rest the injured area until the pain subsides.
- **I**ce: Press a cold compress to the injured area. Do this four to eight times daily, 20 minutes per session.
- **C**ompression: For a minimum of two days, use an elastic compression bandage to support the injured part.
- **E**levation: To reduce swelling, raise the area affected above heart level.

You may need an extra pair of hands if the following conditions arise:

- The person feels severe pain whenever the injured part is moved or touched
- You notice a misshapen or bent limb
- The person feels numbness in the injured area
- Signs of infection such as redness, warmth and swelling are visible

Top Tips to Help You Respond to Emergencies Efficiently

Emergencies can happen when least expected. Of course, that's what makes them emergencies. Keeping the following tips in mind will help you cope:

Don't Panic: Some people panic under pressure. However, remaining calm is one of the most effective ways you can render helpful assistance to whoever needs it.
It's easier not to panic and remain calm if you have prepared in advance for

emergencies. Thus, when you are faced with such challenges, you are well equipped to handle them as professionally.

Check for Bleeding: Are any victims bleeding? If there are, use a clean cloth to apply direct pressure to reduce the bleeding. While at it, don't forget to use protective equipment such as gloves to protect yourself.

Loosen Clothing: Sometimes, too-tight clothing may impede breathing and complicate issues. Thus, you should check for tight clothing and loosen it immediately.

Don't Move Injured Persons: Moving injured people may complicate issues. You may be unaware of internal injuries or fractures which could be worsened by movement. The only time you should move a patient is if he/she is in harm's way, such as in the middle of the road. Patients are best kept quiet and still. You may have to keep them warm if circumstances warrant that.

Call 911 Quickly: Call for assistance without delay. It is advisable that you know emergency numbers by heart or have them in your phone. This may include the number of the ambulance, rescue squad, poison control center or the police.

Check for Fractures: If the patient can't move a part of the body and seems to be in pain, it is likely the individual has suffered a bone fracture. It is not advisable to move the patient. Rather, keep the person motionless unless, as discussed earlier, there is absolutely no other alternative.

Can You be of Help? Whenever you are faced with emergencies, if you have the necessary tools to help, you should render assistance. If not, call more qualified medical personnel to handle the situation. Don't worsen the situation by offering help if you are not able.

Perform CPR: As a medical assistant, you must know CPR. This can be the difference between life and death for a person.

Practice Test 1

1. What is an advance directive?
    a. A source of information for medical workers about the type of treatment that is ideal for a patient
    b. A source of information for medical workers about necessary precautions to take when dealing with contagious diseases
    c. A set of instructions for carrying out necessary tests
    d. A set of instructions for taking samples

2. What is a reference point when making health decisions for terminally ill people?
    a. Living will
    b. Durable power of attorney
    c. Patient Self-Determination Act
    d. None of the above

3. How many physicians must confirm a patient's inability to make personal health decisions before implementing the directives of a living will?
    a. Two
    b. Three
    c. Five
    d. Ten

4. Under which of the following conditions does a patient lose the power to make personal medical decisions?
    a. Being in a coma
    b. Loss of communication ability
    c. Moderate or severe Alzheimer's
    d. All of the above

5. Under what condition is someone considered competent to make personal medical decisions?
    a. The person's memory retention is intact
    b. The person can communicate his/her feelings
    c. All of the above
    d. None of the above

6. Principles of Medical Ethics are divided into how many groups?
    a. Four
    b. Three
    c. Five
    d. Eight

7. What is the principle that requires health-care providers to be cautious of their actions and not pose a threat to their patients?
    a. Principle of patient consideration
    b. Principle of patient-consciousness
    c. Principle of nonmaleficence
    d. Principle of zero threat to patients

8. In which of the following is respect for patients' actions and decisions enshrined?
    a. Principle of consideration
    b. Principle for respect for fundamental human rights
    c. Principle for consideration of patients' health
    d. Principle of respect for autonomy

9. What is the patient exercising when he/she cooperates with the physician's instructions and sticks to a recommended regimen?
    a. Implied consent
    b. Written consent
    c. Inferred consent
    d. Deliberate consent

10. Respect for people's rights and fair distribution of scarce resources are major components of:
    a. Principle of fundamental human rights
    b. Principle of fair distribution
    c. Principle of justice
    d. Principle of equality and equity

11. What is the major component of the Declaration of Helsinki?
    a. Regulation of the activities of the medical community
    b. Regulation of patients' expectations and requests
    c. Regulation of the activities of certified medical assistants
    d. Regulation of the activities of professional surgeons

12. Why is electrical safety important within the medical community?
    a. To reduce the expenses incurred while providing medical care
    b. To reduce patients' exposure to excessive light
    c. To prevent potential accidents that may arise from electrical facilities
    d. All of the above

13. Some of the processes that may increase health-care providers' exposure to radiation are:
    a. X-rays, ultrasounds and CT scans
    b. Ultrasounds and urine sample taking
    c. X-rays and gamma rays
    d. Medical record-keeping and sample storage

14. What is an effective preventive measure against accidentally slipping during cleaning?
    a. Only cleaning on off days
    b. Cleaning a medical facility at night when most patients and staff are asleep
    c. Placing safety signs in appropriate locations
    d. Outsourcing to cleaning firms with years of experience

15. Which of the following are health-care workers immune to?
    a. Biological hazards
    b. Cleaning hazards
    c. Radiation hazards
    d. None of the above

16. Which of the following are important fire and emergency signs?
    a. Muster points and fire exits
    b. Fire extinguishers and water
    c. Fire exits and water
    d. Muster points and entrance points

17. How is ergonomics used?
    a. It highlights the importance of giving a patient appropriate medical care
    b. It ensures medical workers are assigned the right job
    c. It establishes the relationship between a medical worker and a patient
    d. It teaches health-care workers the importance of being dedicated to their work

18. Which of the following medical conditions are occupational hazards for health workers?
    a. Muscle strain and tendonitis
    b. Tendon inflammation and herniated disc
    c. Both A and B
    d. None of the above

19. What are prefixes?
    a. Special terminology for physicians
    b. Special terminology for certified medical assistants
    c. Words added before other words to give them new meaning
    d. Words added after words to give them new meaning

20. What are suffixes?
    a. Special terminology for physicians
    b. Special terminology for certified medical assistants
    c. Words added before other words to give them new meaning
    d. Words added after words to give them new meaning

21. Which of the following is a suffix used for medical terms that express persistent pain in the upper abdomen?
    a. -gnosis
    b. -ectasis
    c. -pepsic
    d. -pepsia

22. Which of the following is a physician who specializes in studying the cause and nature of diseases is?
    a. A pathologist
    b. An allergist or immunologist
    c. A dermatologist
    d. An endocrinologist

23. Which of the following are professionals who specialize in infectious diseases are?
    a. Hematologists
    b. Infectious disease professionals
    c. Infectious disease experts
    d. Infectious disease specialists

24. What are two of the major causes of danger in most medical environments?
    a. Spills and leaks
    b. Sleeping and snoring
    c. Spills and sleeping
    d. Leaks and snoring

25. Which of the following is a factor that determines the most appropriate protective gear for a medical worker is?
    a. The cost of procuring the protective gear
    b. The ease of maintaining the protective gear
    c. The potential harm in different departments
    d. The potential harm patients are exposed to

26. Which of the following is an effective way to increase safety within medical facilities?
    a. Ensuring that all health workers are duly insured
    b. Documenting the cost of purchasing protective gear
    c. Increasing patients' safety knowledge
    d. Charging patients according to their level of exposure to danger

27. People will be more inclined to obey safety guidelines if :
    a. There's a safety compliance plan in place
    b. Brute force is used to ensure compliance with standing orders
    c. They are medicated
    d. Patients who obey are rewarded

28. Which of the following is an accident prevention tip in the workplace?
    a. Having a safety compliance plan in place
    b. Teaching patients safety information
    c. Teaching important safety policies
    d. All of the above

29. A living will can include which of the following?
    a. Whether patients are to be kept alive with ventilators or dialysis machines
    b. Whether patients are willing to accept treatment for certain ailments even if they cannot make such decisions themselves
    c. Whether patients are willing to donate organs after their death
    d. All of the above

30. A legal document that a patient uses to transfer major health-care decisions to a proxy is which of the following?
    a. Durable power of attorney
    b. Consent transfer document
    c. Permanent decision-transfer document
    d. Patient self-determination act document

31. What document should a patient be provided with on admission to a health-care facility?
    a. A document spelling out the facility's policies and the patient's decision-making rights
    b. A document expressing the facility's commitment to caring for patients, irrespective of their status
    c. A document spelling out the terms and conditions under which the patient will be provided with medical services
    d. A legally binding document spelling out the precautionary measure put in place to give patients the best possible treatment

32. What Act was created by the US Congress to amend some previous laws?
    a. The Health Insurance and Accountability Act
    b. The Health Portability Act
    c. The Health Insurance Portability and Accountability Act
    d. The Health Portability and Accountability Act

33. What are two major features of HIPAA?
    a. Portability and renewability
    b. Renewability and flexibility
    c. Flexibility and portability
    d. None of the above

34. What is medical identity theft?
    a. Stealing a medical worker's identity
    b. Using a medical worker's professional tools without consent
    c. Using someone's personal health insurance information fraudulently
    d. Using someone's medical information without permission

35. In order to be valid, consent to treatment must be which of the following?
    a. Voluntary and informed
    b. Informed and well documented
    c. Voluntary and given without undue pressure
    d. Valuable and given without undue pressure

36. A patient expresses his desire to accept any medical treatment. What is this type of consent?
    a. Oral
    b. Implied
    c. Verbal
    d. Written

37. How does the principle of nonmaleficence ensure that health workers pose zero threat or risk to their patients?
    a. By encouraging them to attend only to physically fit patients
    b. By encouraging them to always wear protective equipment
    c. By encouraging them to stick to the best professional standards
    d. By encouraging them to be liberal in their dealings with patients

38. Which is found in the principle of nonmaleficence?
    a. Principle of personal security
    b. Principle of patient's rights
    c. Principle of double effect
    d. Principle of division of labor

39. Which of the following is not a subdivision of the principle of justice?
    a. Respect for acceptable laws
    b. Respect for people's rights
    c. Fair distribution of scarce resources
    d. None of the above

40. A physician/patient privilege governing confidential information a patient shares with his/her physician is covered by which of the following?
    a. The Nuremberg Code
    b. The Declaration of Helsinki
    c. The Hippocratic Oath
    d. The Patient/Physician Oath

41. Which of the following trials were conducted in 1947?
    a. The Nuremberg Medical Tribunals
    b. The Nuremberg Military Tribunals
    c. The Hippocratic Oath Medical Tribunals
    d. The Hippocratic Oath Medical Trials and Tribunals

42. The trial led to the incarceration of how many doctors, while how many were acquitted?
    a. Nine, two
    b. Nine, seven
    c. Seven, nine
    d. Ten, nine

43. Electrical safety can be guaranteed in and around a medical facility through which of the following?
    a. Use of electrode gel and conductive solutions when patients are connected to certain electrical devices
    b. Use of anode gel and electrolytes when patients are connected to electrical devices
    c. Implementation of certain policies to improve security around patients on electrical devices
    d. Implementation of security awareness programs for patients

44. Health-care facilities must comply with the standard set by which of the following to ensure environmental safety?
    a. National Fire Prevention Association
    b. National Fire Control Association
    c. National Fire Protection Association
    d. National Fire Prevention and Control Association

45. What signs are put in strategic places in a medical facility to reduce people's exposure to infectious diseases?
    a. Biohazard signs
    b. Laboratory and biohazard signs
    c. Laboratory and laundry area signs
    d. Cleaning and biohazard signs

46. Which of the following are not common workplace accidents?
    a. Latex allergies, radioactive materials and blood-borne pathogens
    b. Laser danger, back pain and work environment stress
    c. Back pain, blood-borne pathogens and laser danger
    d. None of the above

47. Health-care officials can protect themselves against contact with patients' bodily fluids by:
    a. Taking precautions against blood-borne pathogens
    b. Taking precautions against blood-borne bacteria
    c. Taking precautions against fluid-borne pathogens
    d. Taking precautions against fluid-borne bacteria

48. The suffix used for a wide range of health problems that are caused by the dilation of a body's hollow organ is:
    a. *-ectasis*
    b. *-pepsia*
    c. *-gnosis*
    d. *-lapar*

49. Who is an anesthesiologist?
    a. A medical doctor who specializes in allergies
    b. An expert at numbing pain associated with surgery, childbirth and other painful procedures
    c. A professional at curing painful medical conditions
    d. A specialist in treating pregnant and nursing women

50. Medical conditions associated with the digestive system, such as gallbladder and pancreas problems, are best treated by which of the following?
    a. An endocrinologist
    b. A psychologist
    c. A gastroenterologist
    d. A neurologist

51. What do gynecologists or obstetricians do?
    a. They are specialists who deal with the female reproductive system and other related health conditions
    b. They are specialists in diagnosing and treating patients from infancy through adolescence
    c. They treat infectious diseases like HIV and Lyme disease
    d. They study and discover new ailments

52. What is an appendectomy?
    a. It is a medical procedure performed on people with an inflamed or infected appendix
    b. It is a medical procedure performed on pregnant women
    c. It is a procedure for correcting poor sight
    d. It is a procedure for breast enlargement

53. Differentiate between psoriatic arthritis and rheumatoid arthritis.
    a. Rheumatoid arthritis affects multiple joints simultaneously, while psoriatic arthritis affects psoriasis victims only
    b. Psoriatic arthritis affects multiple joints simultaneously, while rheumatoid arthritis affects teenagers only
    c. Psoriatic arthritis affects adult females, while rheumatoid arthritis is exclusive to adult males
    Rheumatoid arthritis affects infants and adolescents, while psoriatic arthritis affects pregnant women and nursing mothers
54. What does CABG stand for?
    a. Coronary artery battered graft
    b. Coronary artery battered groin
    c. Coronary artery bypass graft
    d. Coronary artery bipedal graft

55. What is a pulmonary embolism?
    a. A medical condition characterized by pain in the groin and lower abdomen
    b. A medical condition characterized by blood clotting in the lungs
    c. A medical condition characterized by blood clotting in the kidneys and lungs
    d. A medical condition that causes abdominal and kidney pains

56. A medical condition that is triggered by either violent shaking of the head or the entire body is called which of the following?
    a. Mild traumatic body injury
    b. Muscular traumatic body infliction
    c. Mild traumatic brain injury
    d. Muscular traumatic brain injury

57. What is type 1 diabetes otherwise known as?
    a. Insulin-defying diabetes mellitus
    b. Insulin-resistant diabetes mellitus
    c. Insulin-responsive diabetes mellitus
    d. Insulin-dependent diabetes mellitus

58. When the body is accidentally attacked by the immune system, the condition is defined as which of the following?
    a. Autoinflammatory body-attacking immune cells
    b. Autoinflammatory reliant immune cells
    c. Autoinflammatory disease
    d. None of the above

59. Lichen sclerosus can be identified by these symptoms:
    a. White spots or patches on the genitals or in the anal areas
    b. White spots or patches at the back and forehead
    c. White spots or patches in the anal areas and behind the neck
    d. White spots or patches on the stomach and the armpits

60. The gynecology profession covers all of the following fields except:
    a. Oncology, reconstructive surgery and surgical operations
    b. Tumor removal and abdominal pain relief
    c. Gynecology and pediatrics
    d. B and C

61. Medical geneticists are professionals who diagnose and treat disorders such as:
    a. Alzheimer's disease and Parkinson's disease
    b. Brain tumors and spinal tumors
    c. Both A and B
    d. None of the above

62. *Oopho-* is a prefix for:
    a. Ovary-related medical conditions
    b. Kidney-related medical conditions
    c. A wide range of ailments that cover both kidney-related and ovary-related diseases
    d. An array of ailments characterized by abdominal pains

63. *Rhino-* is a prefix used for:
    a. A medical condition that affects the lungs and kidneys
    b. A medical condition that affects the lungs and the respiratory tract
    c. A medical condition that affects the nose
    d. A medical condition that can lead to partial blindness and cataracts

64. Why is wiping up considered insufficient for cleaning bodily fluids?
    a. Bodily fluids are slippery
    b. Bodily fluids may contain disease-transmitting bacteria
    c. Bodily fluids can be cleaned only with a concentrated solution
    d. Bodily fluids require urgent cleaning

65. What is the most appropriate protective gear for a medical worker attending to patients suffering from infectious diseases?
    a. Strong gloves and shoes
    b. High-quality masks
    c. Stainless overalls and a pair of goggles
    d. None of the above

66. What effect can a constant reminder have on patients?
    a. They will be more willing to abide by safety rules and regulations
    b. They will understand the importance of following medical advice
    c. They are less likely inclined to handle their medical condition flippantly
    d. All of the above

67. When creating a contingency plan, a medical facility should include all of the following people in the plan except:
    a. Patients
    b. Staff
    c. Visitors
    d. Patients' pets

68. People working in the laundry department of a medical facility are best protected from accidents by wearing which of the following?
    a. Strong gloves
    b. Face masks
    c. Waterproof shoes
    d. None of the above

69. Workplace accidents can lead to serious health issues such as:
    a. Severe coughing
    b. Fractured arms and limbs
    c. Loss of job
    d. Loss of interest in the job

70. Some of the most important effects of placing laboratory and biohazard signs in medical facilities are:
    a. Preventing infectious diseases from spreading across the medical facility
    b. Sensitizing people to the presence of substances that may be injurious to their health
    c. Both A and B
    d. None of the above

71. Where are cleaning and slip hazard signs best placed?
    a. In areas where cleaning has just been completed
    b. In select areas of the medical facility
    c. At the entrance of a medical facility for all visitors and patients to see
    d. In the laundry area

72. When creating awareness about the potential danger of exposure to harmful radiation in a medical facility, the following people should be informed:
    a. Medical staff only
    b. Non-medical staff only
    c. The general public only
    d. The medical teams, members of the public and other hospital staff

73. The living will covers the following medical areas:
    a. Dialysis and life support
    b. Life support and tube feeding
    c. Both A and B
    d. None of the above

74. Which of the following was passed by the United States Congress in 1990?
    a. The Patient Self-Decision Making Act
    b. The Physician Self-Decision Making Act
    c. The Patient Self-Determination Act
    d. The Physician Self-Determination Act

75. What is the full meaning of PSDA?
    a. The Patient Self-Decision Making Act
    b. The Physician Self-Decision Making Act
    c. The Patient Self-Determination Act
    d. The Physician Self-Determination Act

76. Which two laws were amended by the Health Insurance Portability and Accountability Act?
    a. The Employee Retirement Income Security Act and the Public Health Service Act
    b. The Employee Retirement Income Security and Physicians' Ethics Implementation Act
    c. The Public Health Service Act and the Patient Discharge Medical Bills Act
    d. The Employee Retirement Income Security Act and the Medical Services Constitutional Act

77. Which of the following controls information-sharing?
    a. Employee Retirement Act
    b. Patient Discharge Medical Bills Act
    c. Health Insurance Portability and Accountability Act
    d. Information Dissemination and Control Act

78. Which of the following was established by the American Hospital Association in 2003?
    a. Medical Profession Regulatory Body
    b. Patient Care Partnership
    c. Regulatory Body for Patient and Physician Relationship
    d. Medical and Dental Association Regulatory Body

79. Patients have the following responsibilities:
    a. Providing health-care professionals with personal information
    b. Asking relevant questions that may help them to make informed decisions
    c. Making themselves available for appointments
    d. All of the above

80. All information pertaining to treatment must be specifically spelled out according to which of the following kinds of consent?
    a. Informed decision
    b. Emergency situation decision
    c. Informative decision
    d. None of the above

81. Which of the following conditions is not considered when determining whether a patient can make health-care decisions for him/herself?
    a. Ability to pay medical bills
    b. Ability to read and sign documents
    c. Ability to effectively express feelings and decisions through any means of communication
    d. Ability to discern potential hazards and take precautionary measures

82. Under what conditions can a medical worker overrule any form of consent?
    a. If the patient has a serious mental ailment that may impair his/her thinking ability
    b. If the patient has grown-up kids who can make decisions on his/her behalf
    c. If the medical worker is experienced enough to handle whatever medical condition the patient is being treated for
    d. If the medical facility is run by the federal government

83. How many types of consent are there?
    a. Three
    b. Infinite
    c. Ten
    d. Five

84. Which of the following states that patients should be allowed to make personal decisions without having undue pressure placed on them?
    a. The principles of the medical profession
    b. The principles of medical regulations
    c. The principles of medical ethics
    d. The principles of medical instructions

85. This principle addresses medical mistakes.
    a. The principle of respect for autonomy
    b. The principle of medical regulations
    c. The principle of nonmaleficence
    d. The principle of professional instructions

86. Which of the following conditions applies to the principle of nonmaleficence?
    a. An action must not be morally wrong but can be morally neutral
    b. An action may be for the physician's personal interest
    c. An action must be favorable for both patient and physician
    d. An action must be relevant to the existing condition

87. Some factors that influence the principle of justice are:
    a. Sexual preferences and culture
    b. Insurance coverage and place of residence
    c. Sexual preferences and legal capacity
    d. All of the above

88. What defines the principle of double effect?
    a. An action may sometimes have multiple effects
    b. An action may be good and bad simultaneously
    c. An action may have two effects
    d. An action may be both irrelevant and relevant

89. Which of the following is true of the principle of double effect?
    a. The good result must be achieved without resulting in bad side effects
    b. The bad side must outweigh the good side
    c. Both effects must be equal and take place simultaneously
    d. The caregiver must be able to distinguish between the two effects

90. This principle encourages medical workers to promote good actions toward their patients.
    a. The principle of beneficence
    b. The principle of malevolence
    c. The principle of good manners
    d. The principle of professionalism in the medical community

91. Distinguish between the principle of nonmaleficence and the principle of beneficence.
    a. The principle of beneficence stipulates that health-care providers should engage in beneficial actions, while the principle of nonmaleficence requires health-care providers to be cautious of their actions
    b. The principle of nonmaleficence encourages health-care providers to engage in beneficial actions, while the principle of beneficence highlights the need for them to be cautious of their actions
    c. The principle of nonmaleficence applies to medical workers, while the principle of beneficence applies to patients
    d. The principle of beneficence is regulated by the medical community, while the principle of nonmaleficence is regulated by the government

92. Why do some patients have access to good health-care, while others do not?
    a. Factors such as financial status, sexual preference and insurance come into play
    b. Government policies designate the distinction
    c. The medical profession naturally favors some patients over others
    d. Ignorance and illiteracy play a role

93. The Hippocratic Oath was created to:
    a. Establish confidentiality between doctors and their patients
    b. Emphasize the importance of taking medical advice seriously
    c. Show the distinction between a physician and a medical assistant
    d. Regulate both the medical and the dental professions

94. Which of the following medical codes of conduct is superior to any local law?
    a. The Declaration of Hippocratic
    b. The Declaration of Helsinki
    c. The Helsinki Oath
    d. The Hippocratic Oath

95. The Nuremberg Code is based on all of the following except:
    a. Volunteers are needed for experimentation
    b. The benefits of the experiment should outweigh the risks
    c. If there are potentials for injury, disability or death, the experiment should be discontinued
    d. None of the above

96. Moral factors affecting ethical decisions are influenced by:
   a. Cultural values and norms
   b. Local norms and external influences
   c. International and local laws
   d. Environmental and geographical factors

97. Which of the following provide practical alternatives to patient lifting?
   a. Sliding boards, wheelchairs and gait belts
   b. Shower chairs, staircases and electric beds
   c. Sliding boards and staircases
   d. Special beds, wheelchairs and remote-controlled machines

98. What are blood-borne pathogens?
   a. Medical items that can easily pass viruses and bacteria from one person to another
   b. Bodily fluids that serve as virus-transferring mediums
   c. Blood-borne pathogens that transfer viruses and bacteria
   d. Pathogens spread through blood and air

99. What is the benefit of a safety compliance plan?
   a. It enables hospital staff and others to abide by established protocols
   b. It helps individuals understand the existing safety rules
   c. It serves as a constant reminder of the health implications of certain medical treatments
   d. It helps teach safety practices

100. When you teach patients safety information, you are leveraging humans' natural desire to:
   a. Take their health seriously
   b. Contribute meaningfully to whatever will increase their security and safety
   c. None of the above
   d. Both A and B

Practice Test 1 – Answers

1) **a:** A source of information for medical workers about the type of treatment that is ideal for a patient

In recognition of the fact that patients may require different medical treatments, the advance directive provides necessary information that enables medical workers to utilize the most appropriate treatment for a patient. It provides a guideline for unconscious patients or those who lack the mental or physical strength to express themselves.

2) **a:** Living will

When medical workers are faced with making health decisions for terminally ill people, the living will is a reference point that can assist them in making the right decision. It is a legal document that reflects a person's future health-care decisions that physicians can consult when making decisions.

3) **a:** Two

At least two physicians must confirm a patient's inability to make personal health decisions before a living will's content can be considered. This eliminates potential issues that may arise as a result of using the information in the document.

4) **d:** All of the above

A patient may lose the power to make personal medical decisions if he/she is in a coma, has lost the ability to communicate or has any form of Alzheimer's. The onus lies on the physician to decide the best treatment.

5) **c:** All of the above

While a patient's power to decide for him/herself may be removed, the person is in full control of his/her medical care if his/her retentive memory is intact and the person can clearly communicate feelings and decisions.

6) **a:** Four

The principles of medical ethics are divided into four groups. These are the principle of respect for autonomy, the principle of nonmaleficence, the principle of maleficence and the principle of justice.

7) **c:** Principle of nonmaleficence

The principle of nonmaleficence requires health-care providers to exercise caution and ensure that their actions do not pose a threat to patients. Thus, they should desist from any medical practices that will undermine their professionalism and endanger their patients. Rather, they should go out of their way to heal their patients.

8) **d:** Principle of respect for autonomy

This principle contains regulatory guidelines that require health workers to respect their patients' actions and decisions. Thus, each patient should be given the freedom to make health decisions that will impact his/her health unless a patient is not fit to make such decisions.

9) **a:** Implied consent

When a patient cooperates with the treatment instructions, the patient is exhibiting implied consent. When patients willingly submit to using medications and/or to have specimens taken, they also exercise this consent. Such consent is strictly verbal.

10) **c:** Principle of justice

The principle of justice covers some important areas that include respect for people's rights and fair distribution of scarce resources. This implies that patients should not be treated as second-class citizens but should be treated with equality and fairness. Respect for acceptable laws is also enshrined in the principle.

11) **a:** Regulation of the activities of the medical community

The major component of the Declaration of Helsinki is regulation of the activities of the medical community. It contains some ethical principles that guide human experimentation for medical practitioners to ensure their activities are within the boundaries of the medical community and government's ethics.

12) **c:** To prevent potential accidents that may arise from electrical facilities

Modern medical facilities are run on electrical devices. For instance, automated blood pressure cuffs and electric beds are powered by electricity. Thus, electrical safety is important to ensure that patients are not exposed to electrical shocks and other related accidents.

13) **a:** X-rays, ultrasounds and CT scans

When performing these procedures, medical equipment that uses powerful radiation is used. Excessive exposure to the radiation emitted by these pieces of equipment is unhealthy, as it increases patients' vulnerability to radiation-related ailments such as cancer.

14) **c:** Placing safety signs in appropriate places

Accidental slips during cleaning can lead to a wide range of medical conditions, such as sprains, fractured skulls and others. This can be prevented if safety signs are placed in strategic locations to warn people of potential dangers.

15) **d:** None of the above

Health-care workers can be affected by cleaning hazards, radiation hazards and biological hazards.

16) **a:** Muster points and fire exits

Signs and symbols can warn people of dangerous places and help them avoid them. Muster points and fire exits are important too. While the former refers to a safe place where people can converge during a fire, the latter provides a way out of the facility.

17) **b:** It ensures medical workers are assigned the right job

It is imperative that medical workers be assigned duties they are well suited for. This is where ergonomics comes in. It ensures that workers and jobs are not mismatched.

18) **c:** Both A and B

Health workers are exposed to a wide range of health conditions. Tendon inflammation, muscle strain and herniated discs are some of them.

19) **c:** Words added before other words to give them new meaning

Prefixes are words that are put at the beginning of another word to change the meaning. Examples of prefixes are *un-*, *in-*, *im-* and others. For instance, *un* + *able* results in *unable*, changing the meaning of *able.*

20) **d:** Words added after words to give them new meaning

While prefixes are added to the beginning of words to change their meaning, suffixes perform the same function when they are added to the end of words. Some examples are *-pepsia* and *-ectasis*.

21) **d:** *-pepsia*

-pepsia is a suffix used for medical terms that express persistent pain in the upper abdomen. Problems with the digestive tract or indigestion trigger such health conditions. Some examples are propopepsia, bradypepsia, hyperpepsia and oligopepsia.

22) **a:** A pathologist

A pathologist is a physician who deals with the nature and causes of diseases. Pathologists diagnose and monitor diseases through clinical lab tests and microscopic examinations.

23) **d:** Infectious disease specialists

Some medical professionals' area of expertise is treating infectious diseases. Such professionals are known as infectious disease specialists. Pneumonia, HIV/AIDS, Lyme disease and tuberculosis are common infectious diseases.

24) **a:** Spills and leaks

The two major causes of danger in medical facilities are spills and leaks. They can cause hazards, including slips and exposure to harmful substances and chemicals.

25) **c:** The potential harm in different departments

Several factors determine the most appropriate protective gear for a medical worker. One such factor is the potential harm medical workers are exposed to in different departments. For instance, workers in the X-ray and ultrasound department are exposed to radiation, while those in the pharmacy department are not.

26) **c:** Increasing patients' safety knowledge

Safety within a medical facility should not be restricted to health workers. Patients should also be given a sense of responsibility.

27) **a:** There's a safety compliance plan in place

A medical facility can increase people's safety consciousness by having a compliance plan in place. The plan should outline several ways people can ensure their own safety.

28) **d:** All of the above

Accidents in the workplace can be prevented by having a safety compliance plan, enforcing it and teaching patients key safety measures.

29) **d:** All of the above

A patient may consider activating the living will if he/she is considering whether to be kept alive with a dialysis machine or a ventilator, whether to be an organ donor or whether to accept specific medical treatment.

30) **a:** Durable power of attorney

Durable power of attorney is a legal document that patients use to empower a proxy or an agent to make medical decisions on their behalf. It becomes legal and can be activated if patients become incapacitated or are unable to make decisions with respect to their health.

31) **a:** A document spelling out the facility's policies and the patient's decision-making rights

A medical facility should provide a patient with a document that specifically spells out the facility's policies and a patient's decision-making rights. Such information ensures that the patient is kept informed.

32) **c:** The Health Insurance Portability and Accountability Act

The Health Insurance Portability and Accountability Act was enacted by the US Congress to amend previous laws such as the Public Health Service Act (PHSA) and the Employee Retirement Income Security Act (ERISA). HIPAA was enacted to protect people who have health insurance in the United States.

33) **a:** Portability and renewability

The Health Insurance Portability and Accountability Act (HIPAA) offers portable and renewable plans.

34) **c:** Using someone's personal health insurance information fraudulently

Medical identity theft is a criminal offense that involves using someone's personal health information to engage in fraudulent activities, mostly as a way of receiving health-care services that the fraudulent individual ordinarily would not have access to.

35) **a:** Voluntary and informed

A patient is considered to have given consent for a medical treatment under certain conditions. For instance, the patient must do so voluntarily after making an informed decision. Hence, everything about the treatment should be clear to the patient. The patient must not be forced to make the decision.

36) **c:** Verbal

When a patient expresses a desire to accept any medical treatment, the patient is said to have given verbal consent. The doctor can proceed to administer the treatment without breaking any law.

37) **c:** By encouraging them to stick to the best professional standards

The principle of nonmaleficence stipulates that health-care providers should be cautious of their actions. Under no condition must they intentionally pose a threat to their patients, whether deliberately or accidentally.

38) **c:** Principle of double effect

The principle of double effect is embedded in the principle of nonmaleficence. The principle helps us understand that there may be two sides to a coin. An action may have a positive and a negative side. Thus, medical workers should ensure the benefits of a treatment outweigh its cons.

39) **d:** None of the above

The principle of justice has several subdivisions, such as respect for people's rights, respect for acceptable laws and fair distribution of scarce resources. This ensures that patients are not treated based on their economic or social status but on their medical needs.

40) **c:** The Hippocratic Oath

The Hippocratic Oath defines the patient/physician privilege. It stipulates that physicians are forbidden from disclosing confidential information about a patient to a third party unless the information is needed for further treatment or is required to make further medical decisions on behalf of the patient.

41) **b:** The Nuremberg Military Tribunals

The Nuremberg Military Tribunals were conducted in 1947. At the trial, 23 physicians were tried for a wide range of crimes against humanity that they committed during the war. These physicians turned Jewish prisoners into unwilling guinea pigs for various experiments.

42) **b:** Nine, seven

During the trial, nine doctors were found guilty of the criminal charges leveled against them and were convicted. Seven others were found not guilty and were subsequently acquitted. The remaining doctors were given the death penalty.

43) **a:** Use of electrode gel and conductive solutions when patients are connected to certain electrical devices

Several precautionary measures can be put in place to reduce the frequency of accidents related to electrical devices. One such measure is the use of electrode gel and conductive solutions when patients are connected to certain electrical devices.

44) **c:** National Fire Protection Association

The National Fire Protection Association has some rules and regulations that are binding on all medical facilities. One of the rules is that devices that are used for patient care should be properly tested to reduce the risks of electric shock.

45) **b:** Laboratory and biohazard signs

Laboratory and biohazard signs should be placed in strategic areas in a medical facility to create awareness.

46) **d:** None of the above

At the workplace, workers are exposed to a wide range of accidents such as back pain, blood-borne pathogens, radioactive materials and latex allergies.

47) **a:** Taking precautions against blood-borne pathogens

Health-care workers can protect themselves from danger in a couple of ways. An effective preventive measure is taking precautions against blood-borne pathogens. This decreases the risks of contracting diseases through patients' bodily fluids.

48) **a:** *-ectasis*

-ectasis is the suffix used for a wide range of medical conditions that are triggered by the dilation of a body's hollow organ. Examples of medical terms using this suffix are bronchiectasis, esophagectasis and pyopyelectasis.

49) **b:** An expert at numbing pain associated with surgery, childbirth and other painful procedures

Anesthesiologists are medical professionals who administer the appropriate dosage of the right drug to numb pain and make procedures less painful for patients.

50) **c:** A gastroenterologist

A gastroenterologist is a medical professional who treats diseases of the digestive system. Gastroenterologists treat pancreas, stomach and gallbladder problems, along with other problems associated with digestive organs such as abdominal pain, ulcers and jaundice.

51) **a:** They are specialists who deal with the female reproductive system and other related health conditions

An obstetrician or a gynecologist is a medical practitioner who specializes in the female reproductive system. OB-GYNs deal with pregnancy-related issues and address infertility. The profession covers gynecologic care, primary health care for women, oncology and, when necessary, surgical operations.

52) **a:** It is a medical procedure performed on people with an inflamed or infected appendix

An appendectomy is a medical procedure performed on people with an inflamed or infected appendix. The removal of the tube-like part of the bowel is otherwise referred to as an appendicectomy.

53) **a:** Rheumatoid arthritis affects multiple joints simultaneously, while psoriatic arthritis affects psoriasis victims only

Rheumatoid and psoriatic are two types of a medical condition that affects the joints. While psoriatic arthritis affects those with psoriasis, rheumatoid can affect people without a previous history of psoriasis. More so, it can affect multiple joints simultaneously.

54) **c:** Coronary artery bypass graft

A coronary artery bypass graft is a form of surgical operation that is performed on the heart to correct a medical condition.

55) **b:** A medical condition characterized by blood clotting in the lungs

A pulmonary embolism is a medical condition that results in the clotting of the blood in the lungs. Surgery is required to treat the condition.

56) **c:** Mild traumatic brain injury

A mild traumatic brain injury is a medical condition that is triggered by either violent shaking of the head or the entire body.

57) **d :** Insulin-dependent diabetes mellitus

Type 1 diabetes is otherwise known as insulin-dependent diabetes mellitus. It is more difficult to treat than type 2 diabetes. Due to the difficulty of treating this diabetes variant, it can be life-threatening.

58) **c:** Autoinflammatory disease

Autoinflammatory disease refers to a health problem that arises when a body's immune system accidentally attacks the body. The attack can trigger several serious medical conditions, such as fever and joint swelling.

59) **a:** White spots or patches on the genitals or in the anal areas

White spots or patches on the genitals or around the anus are some symptoms of lichen sclerosus. However, some other parts of the body can show these symptoms too. Lichen sclerosus can be painful and lead to itching and bleeding.

60) **d:** A and C

The gynecology profession includes gynecologic care, primary health care for women, oncology, and, when necessary, surgical operations. Gynecologic oncology, reconstructive surgery, reproductive endocrinology, female pelvic medicine and infertility are some other areas in this specialty. However, a gynecologist does not remove tumors or treat abdominal pain.

61) **d:** None of the above

Medical geneticists diagnose and treat disorders that are passed from parents to their children. They do not treat spinal tumors, Alzheimer's disease, brain tumors and Parkinson's disease.

62) **a:** Ovary-related medical conditions

Oopho- is a prefix that is used for ovary-related medical conditions. Some medical terms sharing the prefix are oophoroplasty, oophorrhagia and oophoroplasty.

63) **c:** A medical condition that affects the nose

Rhino- is a prefix for a medical condition that affects the nose. For instance, rhinolalia refers to any defect affecting the nasal passages. Other examples include rhinocele, rhinocephaly and rhinogenous.

64) **b:** Bodily fluids may contain disease-transmitting bacteria

When medical workers come in contact with bodily fluids, they may consider wiping off the fluid. A better alternative is to disinfect the affected area with the right cleaning agent. This is because bodily fluids may contain disease-transmitting bacteria that a simple wipe will not remove.

65) **b:** High-quality masks

The most appropriate protective gear for a medical worker attending to patients being treated for infectious disease is a high-quality mask.

66) **d:** All of the above

When dealing with patients who easily forget appointments or who have the tendency to stop taking their medication halfway through treatment, constant reminders may increase their understanding of the importance of following medical instructions and advice.

67) **d:** Patients' pets

When making safety provisions, a medical facility should consider the patients, medical workers and visitors using the facility. Medical facilities do not make provisions for pets unless they are veterinary clinics.

68) **a:** Strong gloves

People working in the laundry department of a medical facility should always wear sturdy gloves when working. The gloves will protect them against accidental wounds that may be caused by sharp objects such as needles.

69) **b:** Fractured limbs

Slipping and falls can lead to fractured limbs at the workplace. Other types of accidents, such as radiation exposure, can also trigger medical conditions.

70) **c:** Both A and B

Some important effects of placing laboratory and biohazard signs in medical facilities are to sensitize people to the presence of potentially injurious substances and prevent infectious disease from spreading from one part of the facility to another.

71) **a:** In areas where cleaning has just been completed

Cleaning and slip hazard signs are best placed in areas where cleaning is done. The signs warn people to take necessary precautions that will prevent them from falling when walking in such areas.

72) **d:** The medical teams, members of the public and other hospital staff

When creating awareness about the potential dangers of exposure to harmful radiation in a medical facility, medical staff, patients and other hospital staff using the facility should be advised.

73) **c:** Both A and B

The living will covers a patient's medical decisions on life support and dialysis. It also addresses decisions relating to tube feeding and using CPR.

74) **c:** The Patient Self-Determination Act

The Patient Self-Determination Act was passed by the United States Congress in 1990. The legislation made it mandatory for health agencies, such as nursing homes, hospitals, home health agencies and other health-care providers, to give adult patients sufficient information about existing advance health-care directives.

75) **c:** The Patient Self-Determination Act

PSDA means Patient Self-Determination Act. This act empowers patients to have access to every piece of information about them. Medical facilities are under obligation to provide such information at will.

76) **a:** The Employee Retirement Income Security Act and the Public Health Service Act

The Health Insurance Portability and Accountability Act was enacted to block some loopholes in previous laws, such as the Public Health and Accountability Act and the Employee Retirement Income Security Act.

77) **c:** The Health Insurance Portability and Accountability Act

Information-sharing within the medical profession is controlled by the Health Insurance Portability and Accountability Act. The act governs how patients' information is used and shared. This is an attempt to ensure that patients' personal medical data is properly protected.

78) **b:** Patient Care Partnership

The American Hospital Association created the Patient Care Partnership in 2003 to help patients have a balanced view of their expectations and responsibilities when receiving treatment in a health-care facility.

79) **d:** All of the above

A patient has several responsibilities, including furnishing physicians with personal information that will prove helpful when providing treatment, asking questions when necessary and keeping up with appointments.

80) **a:** Informed decision

All information pertaining to a treatment must be specifically spelled out according to informed consent. This is to prevent ambiguity of consent and the consequences of any misinterpretation of consent that may arise if the consent is not fully expressed in clear and understandable terms.

81) **a:** Ability to pay medical bills

When determining whether patients can make health-care decisions for themselves, several factors are taken into consideration. Ability to read and sign documents, the ability to clearly express feelings and communicate decisions, and the ability to identify potential hazards and take precautionary measures against them are considered.

82) **a:** If the patient has a serious mental ailment that may impair his/her thinking ability

A physician can overrule any form of consent if the patient has a serious mental ailment, such as dementia, bipolar disorder or schizophrenia, that may impair his/her thinking ability. A physician does not need any form of consent before treating a patient living in an environment that may further worsen his/her condition.

83) **a:** Three

There are three types of consent: written consent, implied consent and verbal consent. Physicians require any form of consent from a patient before treatment. Some exceptions are when a patient is indisposed or living in dangerous conditions.

84) **c:** The principles of medical ethics

The principles of medical ethics state that patients should be allowed to make personal medical decisions without being put under unnecessary pressure. They should make informed and voluntary decisions.

85) **c:** The principle of nonmaleficence

The principle of nonmaleficence takes into account medical mistakes. The goal is to ensure that such mistakes don't pose a big threat to a patient's health or life. Patients' safety and security must be prioritized. Thus, physicians should ensure that a treatment option offers more benefits than side effects.

86) **a:** An action must not be morally wrong but can be morally neutral

One of the conditions that apply to the principle of nonmaleficence is that a medical procedure must not be morally wrong to be considered okay for implementation; it must be morally neutral. Also, the benefits must outweigh the side effects.

87) **d:** All of the above

The principle of justice is influenced by some factors, such as insurance coverage, legal capacity, place of residence and sexual preference. It is not uncommon for wealthy people to get the best available medical treatment, while individuals with fewer resources may be deprived of such high-quality treatment.

88) **c:** An action may have two effects

The underlying principle behind the principle of double effect is that an action may not be totally bad or good. However, a doctor should not consider a medical procedure whose cons outweigh the pros.

89) **a:** The good result must be achieved without resulting in bad effects

The principle of double effect accepts that every good treatment may have a side effect. However, the principle stipulates that the good result of a treatment should not be determined by its side effects. More so, the bad effect must be insignificant in comparison to the good results.

90) **a:** The principle of beneficence

The principle of beneficence encourages medical workers to promote beneficent actions toward their patients. Thus, they must do everything possible to ensure their patients' safety and security. Medical health practitioners are required by this principle to always impact their patients positively.

91) **a:** The principle of beneficence stipulates that health-care providers should engage in beneficial actions, while the principle of nonmaleficence requires health-care providers to be cautious of their actions

While both the principle of beneficence and the principle of nonmaleficence were created to establish good relationships between patients and their physicians, the former promotes beneficent actions toward patients, while the latter encourages health-care workers to be cautious of their actions.

92) **a:** Factors such as financial status, sexual preference and insurance come into play

Several factors play a major role in the disparity in the type and quality of medical care a patient may have access to. Some of these factors are financial status, insurance and sexual preference. This explains why the best medical care is accessible to some people and inaccessible to others.

93) **a:** Establish confidentiality between doctors and their patients

The Hippocratic Oath was created to establish confidentiality between doctors and their patients. It is the foundation for several other guiding rules and principles, which include the principle of nonmaleficence and medical confidentiality. The primary objective is to ensure that patients' secrets are safe with their physicians.

94) **b:** The Declaration of Helsinki

The Declaration of Helsinki is a medical code of conduct that is superior to any local or international law. It contains ethical principles that guide human experimentation. It is morally binding on everyone in the medical field.

95) **d:** None of the above

The Nuremberg Code ensures that only volunteers are used for experimentation. More so, an experiment must be discontinued if it poses a threat to the life of a volunteer or may cause an injury. The risks of the experiment should pale in comparison to the benefits.

96) **a:** Cultural values and norms

Ethical decisions are affected by cultural values and norms, among other factors. External influences, international laws, environmental factors and geographical factors have zero impact on such decisions.

97) **a:** Sliding boards, wheelchairs and gait belts

Health workers are advised to lift patients only when there are no alternatives. Rather, they are encouraged to use object-lifting equipment, such as wheelchairs, sliding boards and gait belts, as a way to lessen their vulnerability to accidents when lifting patients.

98) **c:** Blood-borne pathogens that transfer viruses and bacteria

Medical workers may be infected with diseases during the course of their work. One major means of such infection is through blood-borne pathogens that carry viruses and bacteria.

99) **a:** It enables hospital staff and others to abide by established protocols

One of the benefits of the Safety Compliance Plan is that it enables hospital staff and others to abide by established safety procedures that reduce their vulnerability to accidents and other things that may undermine their safety.

100) **d:** Both A and B

When patients are taught safety information, you are leveraging their desire to be healthy, take their health seriously and contribute meaningfully to whatever will make them safer.

Practice Test 2

1. Why is the medical profession regulated?
    a. To ensure it has the right number of workers
    b. To maintain a good physician/patient ratio
    c. To ensure it meets its goal of meeting people's medical needs legally
    d. To give the profession its deserved recognition

2. Which of the following enables individuals to make adequate preparations for their health, especially when they are unconscious or lack the power to decide for themselves?
    a. Living will
    b. Durable power of attorney
    c. Power of decision-making for indisposed people
    d. Durable power of physicians and attorney

3. Patients find the durable power of attorney useful when:
    a. They wish to transfer their properties to their next of kin
    b. They are concerned about their health
    c. They wish to transfer their health-care decisions to an agent or proxy
    d. They are preparing their will

4. Which of the following is not covered by the Patient Self-Determination Act?
    a. The right to make health-care decisions
    b. The right to choose whatever form of medical treatment a person does or does not want
    c. The right to opt for an advance health-care directive
    d. The right to determine how long a person will accept a medical treatment

5. What does an otolaryngologist specialize in?
    a. Medical disorders in the sinuses, nose and throat
    b. Medical conditions in the urinary tract
    c. Medical challenges such as bipolar disorder
    d. Body weaknesses and pain in the bones and joints

6. The technique used by medical facilities to gather information about clients for clinical analysis is:
    a. Diagnostic analysis
    b. Diagnostic data harvesting
    c. Diagnostic data collection
    d. Diagnostic testing
7. What is a major benefit of the Health Insurance Portability and Accountability Act?
    a. A reduction in the number of older patients
    b. A reduction in pregnancy rates among teenagers
    c. A reduction in identity theft within medical circles
    d. A reduction in the number of medical workers going into the insurance field

8. HIPAA's impact can be felt in all of the following areas of the medical profession except:
    a. Health-care billing services and policies
    b. Increasing hospital fees
    c. Health policies and record-keeping
    d. Specimen collection and accident prevention

9. Differentiate between a psychiatrist and a gastroenterologist.
    a. A psychiatrist treats mental problems, while a gastroenterologist treats issues with the digestive system
    b. A psychiatrist treats mental problems, while a gastroenterologist treats issues with the reproductive system
    c. A psychiatrist treats mental problems, while a gastroenterologist treats issues with the urinary system
    d. A psychiatrist treats mental problems, while a gastroenterologist treats issues with the central nervous system

10. Patients' rights to express their feelings and concerns are expressed in which of the following?
    a. Patient's Freedom of Choice and Expression
    b. Patient's Bills of Rights
    c. Patient's Care and Expressions Right
    d. Patient's Freedom of Expression and Choice

11. The Patient Care Partnership includes all of the following, which patients are entitled to, except:
    a. A safe environment
    b. A clean environment
    c. Optimum protection of privacy
    d. Free medical care

12. Before treating a patient, a medical worker must seek the patient's consent through which of the following?
    a. Consent to medical attention
    b. Consent to specimen collection
    c. Consent to treatment
    d. Consent to information collection

13. In the absence of a durable power of attorney for a patient who cannot make medical decisions, a physician can proceed with the treatment provided that which of the following is true?
    a. The patient has grown-up kids
    a. The patient can pay the medical bills
    b. The patient is still alive
    c. The treatment will serve the patient's interest

14. Define appendectomy.
    a. An appendectomy is a medical procedure that involves the removal of a bad limb through a surgical operation
    b. An appendectomy is a medical procedure that involves altering the abdomen's shape through a surgical operation
    c. An appendectomy is a medical procedure that involves the removal of an inflamed or infected appendix through a surgical operation
    d. An appendectomy is a medical procedure that involves the treatment of an infected appendix

15. What form of consent is needed if a physician wants to attend to a patient living in unsanitary conditions?
    a. Consent of evacuation
    b. Consent of immediate treatment
    c. Consent of treatment
    d. No consent

16. Differentiate between a Source-Oriented Medical Record and a Problem-Oriented Medical Record.
    a. A Problem-Oriented Medical Record contains information about a patient's health status, while a Source-Oriented Medical Record is a data-recording format
    b. A Source-Oriented Medical Record contains information about a patient's health status, while a Problem-Oriented Medical Record is a data-recording format
    c. A Problem-Oriented Medical Record contains information about a patient's financial status, while a Source-Oriented Medical Record contains information about the patient's health status
    d. A Problem-Oriented Medical Record contains information about a patient's medical history, while a Source-Oriented Medical Record contains information about a patient's work history

17. Who makes medical decisions for minors?
    a. The minors can make those decisions
    b. Parents can make such decisions on behalf of minors
    c. The physician can make decisions on behalf of patients who are minors
    d. The government has the responsibility of making such decisions

18. What are medical ethics?
    a. A set of moral principles guiding new medical staff
    b. A set of moral principles for nursing students
    c. A set of moral values regulating the activities of medical practitioners
    d. A set of rules guiding the relationship between patients and physicians

19. That cause and action must be proportional to each other is one of the tenets of which of the following?
    a. The principle of beneficence
    b. The principle of nonmaleficence
    c. The principle of double effect
    d. The principle of action and reaction

20. Which record is created to monitor a patient's progress?
    a. Monitoring and Progress Notes
    b. Monitoring Notes
    c. Medical Information and Monitoring Notes
    d. Progress Notes

21. Informed consent is a concept based upon which of the following?
    a. The principle of beneficence
    b. The principle of nonmaleficence
    c. The principle of respect for autonomy
    d. The principle of action and reaction

22. Who were the majority of people tried under the Nuremberg Code?
    a. Physicians who committed crimes against humanity during World War II
    b. Physicians who committed crimes against humanity during World War I
    c. Physicians who committed crimes against humanity during the Korean War
    d. Physicians who committed crimes against humanity during the Vietnam War

23. Define Personal Identifying Information.
    a. Information about a patient's medical history
    b. Information a patient must provide a medical facility before being attended to
    c. Confidential information about a patient
    d. All of the above

24. What led to the creation of the Nuremberg Code?
    a. It was created to address the issue of doctors who reportedly committed crimes during World War II
    b. The government saw the need to regulate the activities of medical practitioners
    c. The profession needed recognition
    d. The code was a response to a call for medical practitioners to have an umbrella body

25. A list of the electrical equipment used in a medical facility includes all of the following except:
    a. Defibrillation pads
    b. Ultrasound equipment
    c. Patient monitors
    d. Lawn mowers

26. The following are two factors that make safety symbols and signs important for medical workers.
    a. Ease of exposure to hazardous substances and insufficient rest
    b. Insufficient rest and poor wages
    c. Ease of exposure to hazardous substances and nature of their work
    d. Nature of their work and poor wages

27. Some procedures that can emit powerful radiation in hospitals are:
    a. X-rays and CT scans
    b. Ultrasounds and CT scans
    c. CT scans and X-rays
    d. All of the above

28. What are the possible consequences of a fire in a medical facility?
    a. Destruction of property and medical equipment
    b. Panic and confusion
    c. Loss of life
    d. All of the above

29. Which of these records contains information received from a patient before admission?
    a. Nursing Assistant Note
    b. Problem-Oriented Medical Record
    c. History and Physical
    d. Progress and Information Notes

30. Aside from exposure to radiation, what other accidents may occur in a hospital?
    a. Falls or slips
    b. Work environment stress
    c. Both A and B
    d. None of the above

31. Who is a geriatric medicine specialist?
    a. A medical professional who specializes in treating ailments in adult males
    b. A medical professional who specializes in treating ailments in adult females
    c. A medical professional who specializes in treating ailments in adult sports professionals
    d. A medical professional who specializes in treating ailments in the elderly

32. One of the most common ways medical workers are exposed to infections is through:
    a. Sneezing and coughing
    b. Coming into contact with patients' bodily fluids
    c. Exposure to radioactive substances
    d. Slips or falls

33. Which of these people should be excluded from safety awareness in a medical facility?
    a. Medical team
    b. Other members of staff
    c. Patients and their relatives
    d. No one should be exempted

34. Protective equipment protects a medical worker against which of the following?
    a. Bodily damage resulting from falls or slips
    b. Infection through contact with a patient's bodily fluids
    c. Both A and B
    d. None of the above

35. Differentiate between *ultra-* and *ante-*.
    a. *Ante-* means in front of or before, while *ultra-* means beyond or excessive
    b. *Ante-* means beyond or excessive, while *ultra-* means before or in front of
    c. *Ante-* means black, while *ultra-* means white
    d. *Ante-* means tiny or small, while *ultra-* means big or plentiful

36. *Osseo-* and *arthro-* are prefixes used for which of the following?
    a. Bone joints, bones
    b. Bones, bone joints
    c. Breast, milk
    d. Milk, breast

37. What do medical practitioners have access to that assists them in using patients' medical records?
    a. Four charts
    b. Five charts
    c. Three charts
    d. Two charts

38. The prefix used for all nasal medical conditions is:
    a. *Gastr-*
    b. *Bi-*
    c. *Rhino-*
    d. *Colpo-*

39. Who is an ophthalmologist?
    a. A medical expert who specializes in treating eye diseases
    b. A medical expert who specializes in treating nose and ear diseases
    c. A medical expert who specializes in treating pregnancy-related ailments
    d. A medical expert who specializes in treating kidney ailments

40. Medical experts who specialize in treating diabetes, infertility and thyroid problems are:
    a. Gastroenterologists
    b. Endocrinologists
    c. Dermatologists
    d. Cardiologists

41. A surgical procedure that helps people with weight problems is:
    a. Breast augmentation or implants
    b. Abdominoplasty
    c. Gastric bypass surgery
    d. Fat removal surgery

42. Define alopecia areata.
    a. A medical condition that causes swelling and pain in some body parts
    b. A medical condition characterized by hair loss or balding
    c. A medical condition that results in stunted growth
    d. A medical condition peculiar to adults

43. What is epidermolysis bullosa?
    a. A medical problem that affects the bones and bone joints
    b. A medical condition that affects the skin
    c. A medical condition known for causing pain and swelling in the stomach
    d. A group of diseases that cause painful blisters on the skin

44. A medical condition that is characterized by respiratory failure is:
    a. Atherosclerotic cardiovascular disease
    b. Insulin-dependent diabetes mellitus
    c. Acute respiratory distress syndrome
    d. Anterior cruciate ligament failure

45. Which of the following is needed when at least two physicians are treating a patient?
    a. Problem-Oriented Medical Record
    b. Source-Oriented Medical Record
    c. Source-Organized Medical Record
    d. Problem-Organized Medical Record

46. Which of the following medical conditions is otherwise known as a concussion?
    a. Mild traumatic brain infection
    b. Multifaceted traumatic brain injury
    c. Mild traumatic brain injury
    d. Multifaceted traumatic brain infection

47. A medical professional who can handle surgical breast repairs and skin repairs is known as which of the following?
    a. Plastic surgeon
    b. Human body surgeon
    c. Iron surgeon
    d. Professional body repair expert

48. Under which of the following conditions can a patient consider using a living will?
    a. If the patient will accept IV feeding or hydration as necessary
    b. If a patient can pay his/her medical bills
    c. If a patient can transfer the power of attorney to the medical team or family members
    d. If a patient can give written or oral consent for any form of treatment

49. Which of the following is a major factor considered when choosing a proxy for a power of attorney?
    a. The financial status of the potential proxy candidate
    b. The relationship between the potential proxy candidate and the patient
    c. The profession of the potential proxy candidate
    d. The distance between the potential proxy candidate and the medical facility

50. A woman who cannot conceive naturally and wants children should consult which of the following?
    a. A child-rearing expert
    b. A sexologist
    c. A gynecologist or an obstetrician
    d. A professor of the female reproductive system

51. Which of the following is a very important factor to consider when deciding to use a durable power of attorney?
    a. State of residence
    b. Medical history
    c. Monthly income and expenses.
    d. How long a patient has been managing a chronic ailment

52. The objective of the Patient Self-Determination Act is to ensure that:
    a. Patients are familiar with the operations of the medical workers
    b. Patients are able to determine if they should seek medical assistance or not
    c. Patients are not kept in the dark about their health
    d. Patients are well prepared in advance for any medical assistance they may need

53. Patients with all of the following medical conditions except which may lose their power to make medical decisions?
    a. A persistent vegetative state
    b. Kidney failure
    c. Coma
    d. Someone who has recently lost their home

54. Which of the following is not a POMR benefit?
    a. It makes the documenting of chronic illnesses easier
    b. It helps physicians when treating multiple illnesses simultaneously
    c. It helps patients to have better knowledge of their condition
    d. It helps patients decide where to be treated

55. The discharge summary is which of the following?
    a. An official letter written to relieve a physician of his/her job
    b. A letter written to call non-medical staff to order
    c. A document written to discharge a patient from a hospital at the completion of treatment
    d. A document signed by a hospital chief medical director

56. Noncompliance with the Health Insurance Portability and Accountability Act is considered:
    a. A personal decision
    b. A decision that is dependent on a wide range of factors
    c. Excusable under some extenuating circumstances
    d. A criminal offense

57. Under what conditions can the information provided in HIPAA be disclosed?
    a. As required by the law
    b. To prevent a threat to the patient's health or safety
    c. To show the superiority of the medical profession over patients
    d. When a patient is in a vegetative state

58. What did Dr. Lawrence Weed introduce in the 1950s?
    a. Problem-Oriented Medical Record
    b. Source-Oriented Medical Record
    c. Source-Organized Medical Record
    d. Problem-Organized Medical Record

59. What does the Patient Care Partnership address?
    a. It addresses patients' medical history
    b. It addresses patients' income and ability to receive the best care
    c. It considers patients' responsibilities and rights when receiving medical care
    d. It gives health workers insight into patients' minds

60. Which of the following is not included in the Patient's Bill of Rights?
    a. How patients can have access to excellent hospital care
    b. How patients can have a say in their own care
    c. How patients can enjoy medical care in a safe and clean environment
    d. How patients can dictate the medical treatment they accept or reject

61. What is a medical record?
    a. It is a record of the medical staff of a hospital
    b. It is a record of non-medical staff of a medical facility
    c. It is a record of the patients in a medical facility
    d. It is a record of both the medical workers and non-medical staff of a health facility

62. In what ways can patients be involved in their own medical care?
    a. They must be involved in the decision-making process
    b. They can accept or reject any medical treatment
    c. They should know the pros and cons of each medical treatment option they can choose from
    d. All of the above

63. Which of the following is not a subsection of SOMR?
    a. Nursing/Medical Assisting Notes
    b. Diagnostic Testing
    c. History and Physical
    d. Fundamental and Basic

64. Which is not a patient's responsibility?
    a. Providing health-care services with important personal information that will result in better treatment
    b. Asking relevant questions that can assist them in making informed medical decisions
    c. Notifying the medical team in advance if they must cancel an appointment
    d. Informing the medical team of their financial status ahead of any medical treatment for billing purposes

65. Which of the following medical laws is considered part of international human rights law?
    a. The Hippocratic Oath
    b. The Declaration of Helsinki
    c. The Nuremberg Code
    d. Consent to Treatment

66. All of the following are branches of pediatrics except:
    a. Pediatric endocrinology
    b. Adolescent medicine
    c. Pediatric cardiology
    d. None of the above

67. What is the full meaning of SOMR?
    a. Scientific Ordinance Medical Record
    b. Specific Organization Medical Record
    c. Source-Oriented Medical Record
    d. Source-Organized Medical Record

68. Two conditions that must be satisfied for consent to treatment are:
    a. The consent must be voluntary
    b. The patient must make an informed decision
    c. Both A and B
    d. None of the above

69. What is hidradenitis suppurativa?
    a. It is a medical condition with low blood pressure and high body temperature as symptoms
    b. It is a medical condition with pimple-like bumps and boils as symptoms
    c. It is a medical condition with low blood pressure and high body temperature as symptoms
    d. It is a medical condition with low blood pressure and blisters as symptoms

70. How many conditions must be met before a patient is considered to have the ability to make medical decisions for him/herself?
    a. Four
    b. Five
    c. Six
    d. Ten

71. A document containing important data about a patient's condition is called which of the following?
    a. A medical record
    b. A flow sheet
    c. A personal profile sheet
    d. None of the above

72. Surgery requires what kind of consent?
    a. Oral
    b. Written
    c. Virtual
    d. Implied

73. Which of the following is not an example of implied consent?
    a. Blood-sample taking
    b. Blood pressure testing
    c. Using medications
    d. A document signed for a surgical procedure

74. Pediatricians specialize in which of the following?
    a. Performing surgical operations to remove brain tumors
    b. Repairing damaged parts of the body through surgical operations
    c. Treating ailments common to infants through adolescents
    d. Treating ailments common to nursing mothers

75. Factors that influence some medical practitioners' attitudes toward patients are:
    a. Racism and poverty
    b. Sexism and prejudice
    c. Poverty and prejudice
    d. All of the above

76. Which of the following is not a medical code of conduct?
    a. The Hippocratic Oath
    b. The Hippocratic Allegiance and Regulatory Oath
    c. The Declaration of Helsinki
    d. The Nuremberg Code

77. What three things does fire need to become active?
    a. A source of ignition, a source of fuel and oxygen
    b. A source of ignition, a source of water and oxygen
    c. Both A and B
    d. None of the above

78. To prevent electrical hazards, medical facilities should test their electrical devices on which of the following?
    a. Cloud-hosted testing systems
    b. Grounded power devices
    c. Special mechanical and electrical testing devices
    d. Grounded power systems

79. What is clinical correspondence?
    a. Information about a patient sent to a doctor or received by a doctor
    b. Information sent between nurses and doctors
    c. Information sent between doctors only
    d. Information sent between nurses only

80. Reddened skin and pimples are symptoms of:
    a. Psoriatic arthritis
    b. Rosacea
    c. Spinal stenosis
    d. Sports injuries

81. What does OSHA Standard 1910 do to guarantee environmental safety?
    a. Makes a list of work practices and grounding requirements for medical facilities
    b. Makes it compulsory for all medical workers to undergo safety training
    c. Recommends annual training for top physicians
    d. Restricts the construction of medical facilities to certain geographical locations

82. Which of the following is not an effective workplace accident prevention measure?
    a. Taking precautions against blood-borne pathogens
    b. Teaching important safety policies
    c. Having a safety compliance plan in place
    d. Reducing the number of health workers to prevent overcrowding

83. What are two components of the Safety and Health Management System?
    a. Using protective equipment and reporting hazards immediately
    b. Reporting hazards and sheltering in place
    c. Using protective equipment and staying in place
    d. All of the above

84. Differentiate between *micro-* and *lacto-*.
    a. *Lacto-* is a prefix for milk, while *micro-* means small or tiny
    b. *Micro-* means milk, while *lacto-* is a prefix for small or tiny
    c. Both terms can be used interchangeably
    d. They are antonyms

85. Define tendinitis.
    a. A medical condition characterized by constant headaches
    b. A medical condition characterized by high fever
    c. A medical condition characterized by swelling and pain in the joints
    d. A medical condition characterized by constant headaches

86. Which of the following are not medical prefixes?
    a. *Intra-* and *osseo-*
    b. *Micro-* and *lacto-*
    c. *Melan-* and *ante-*
    d. None of the above

87. Identify the odd words in the options below:
    a. *-gnosis* and *-itis*
    b. *-ectasis* and *rhino-*
    c. *Lapar-* and *pathologists*
    d. *Cardiologist* and *ophthalmologist*

88. Ailments associated with the muscle tissue use the following prefix:
    a. *Myo-*
    b. *Oophor-*
    c. *Lapar-*
    d. *Colpo-*

89. Food allergies and insect sting allergies are treated by specialists known as:
    a. Ophthalmologists
    b. Pathologists
    c. Immunologists
    d. Dermatologists

90. Who are neurologists?
    a. Medical professionals who treat hormones and metabolism issues
    b. Medical professionals who handle kidney-related medical conditions
    c. Specialists who treat issues with the nervous system
    d. Specialists who perform surgical operations on the nervous system

91. Psychiatrists are trained to do which of the following?
    a. Identify and treat the causes of infertility
    b. Treat sexually-transmitted diseases and infections
    c. Understand the connection between people's emotions and their mental health
    d. Treat abdominal pain and cancers of the digestive organs

92. Internists are medical professionals who do which of the following?
    a. Treat people with emotional and mental problems
    b. Identify the sources and nature of ailments
    c. Treat diseases affecting the internal organs
    d. Treat medical conditions that are peculiar to infants and adolescents

93. Which of the following medical professionals treat issues with the spinal cord, Parkinson's disease and Alzheimer's disease?
    a. Medical geneticists
    b. Infectious disease specialists
    c. Otolaryngologists
    d. Neurologists

94. What is an operative note?
    a. It is a report about a patient written in his/her medical record after a surgical operation
    b. It is a record of the activities of a patient while taking his/her blood sample
    c. It is a report of the interactive session between a patient and a physician
    d. It is a report of the multiple treatment options a patient can choose from

95. Which of the following is helpful when treating a patient with complex medical conditions?
    a. POMR
    b. SROM
    c. HISPAA
    d. PROMS

96. Where is the larger part of the heart?
    a. Toward the right side of the midline
    b. Below the midline
    c. Toward the left side of the midline
    d. Above the midline

97. Liver failure can be caused by which of the following?
    a. Excessive alcohol consumption and genetic diseases
    b. Consumption of sugar-rich drinks and food
    c. Genetic diseases and overeating
    d. Dehydration and overeating

98. The female reproductive system is divided into which two parts?

a. Simple and complex organs
b. Internal and external organs
c. Primary and secondary organs
d. Left and right organs

99. What are the two major parts of the penis?

a. The shaft and the glans
b. The opening and the head
c. The head and the glans
d. The shaft and the head

100. Which of the following plays an important role when scheduling appointments?

a. Late patients
b. Patients' personal needs
c. Physicians' preferences
d. All of the above

Practice Test 2 – Answers

1) **c:** To ensure it meets its goal of meeting people's medical needs legally.

The medical profession, like every other profession, is regulated. The primary objective is to ensure that medical workers meet people's medical needs within the confines of the law.

2) **a:** Living will

The living will enables individuals to make adequate preparation for their health care, especially when they have a serious ailment or are unconscious and, therefore, cannot make decisions for themselves.

3) **c:** They wish to transfer their health-care decisions to an agent or proxy

The durable power of attorney is a powerful document that can enable a sick person to make some decisions through a proxy or agent.

4) **d:** The right to determine how long a person will accept a medical treatment

The Patient Self-Determination Act addresses several issues. One of them is a patient's right to determine how long he/she is willing to accept medical treatment. It also addresses a patient's right to accept or refuse treatment and the right to opt for an advanced health-care directive.

5) **a:** Medical disorders in the sinuses, nose and throat

Physicians specialize in different subsections of medicine. An otolaryngologist handles medical conditions that specifically affect the nose, sinuses and throat.

6) **d:** Diagnostic testing

Diagnostic testing is used by medical facilities to gather necessary information from their patients for clinical analysis. Some specimens that are collected include sputum, blood and urine.

7) **c:** A reduction in identity theft within medical circles

The medical community is not immune to identity theft. To reduce identity theft, the Health Insurance Portability and Accountability Act was enacted.

8) **b:** Increasing hospital fees

HIPAA's impact can be felt in some areas, such as accident prevention and specimen collection. It is also useful in health-care billing services, record-keeping at health insurance companies and in other medical areas.

9) **a:** A psychiatrist treats mental problems, while a gastroenterologist treats issues with the digestive system

While a gastroenterologist is an expert in issues related to the digestive system, a psychiatrist handles mental problems.

10) **b:** Patient's Bill of Rights

The Patient's Bill of Rights empowers patients to express their feelings and reservations about medical treatments. They are also entitled to answers to their questions, provided such answers will make a positive impact on their health or the type of treatment they can accept or reject.

11) **d:** Free medical care

According to the Patient Care Partnership, patients are entitled to a safe medical environment that is clean and poses no threat to their health. The medical facility must also offer optimum protection of privacy. It does not offer free medical care for patients.

12) **c:** Consent to treatment

Before performing any treatment, it is mandatory that a physician obtain consent from patients. The consent may be given orally, put down in writing or implied through the patient's actions. No treatment should commence without this consent.

13) **c:** The treatment will serve the patient's interest

When a patient is in a vegetative state and has lost the ability to make decisions, durable power of attorney can speak for the person. However, in the absence of durable power of attorney, a physician can exercise his/her authority and proceed with any treatment that will benefit the patient.

14) **c:** An appendectomy is a medical procedure that involves the removal of the inflamed or infected appendix through a surgical operation

An appendectomy focuses on removing a patient's inflamed or infected appendix surgically.

15) **d:** No consent

Although a physician must obtain consent from a patient before proceeding with any medical treatment, there are exceptions to the rule. One of the exceptions is that a physician does not need such consent if the patient lives in an unhygienic environment that may further harm the person's health.

16) **a:** A Problem-Oriented Medical Record contains information about a patient's health status, while a Source-Oriented Medical Record is a data-recording format

While both Problem-Oriented Medical Records and Source-Oriented Medical Records are procedures that are associated with medical records, the former contains information about a patient's health status, while the latter is a data-recording format.

17) **b:** Parents can make such decisions on behalf of minors

While individuals are responsible for making their own medical decisions, especially if they are mentally and physically able to do so, minors cannot do so. Their parents must decide for them.

18) **c:** A set of moral values regulating the activities of medical practitioners

Medical ethics are designed to regulate the medical profession and ensure that medical workers are not going beyond their boundaries while discharging their duties.

19) **c:** The principle of double effect

One of the fundamentals of the principle of double effect is that a cause and action must be proportional to each other. This implies that medical practitioners must give a patient proportional medical treatment for an ailment.

20) **d:** Progress Notes

Progress notes are some important components of a patient's medical record. This sheet serves as a basis for health-care professionals to record the clinical status of a patient.

21) **c:** The principle of respect for autonomy

The health-care profession, through the principle of respect for autonomy, guarantees total respect for patients' decisions and actions. This implies that patients should be given the freedom to make decisions that will impact their health.

22) **a:** Physicians who committed crimes against humanity during World War II

The Nuremberg Code was created in 1947 to try some physicians who perpetrated all sorts of crimes against humanity during WWII. Some of the physicians were found guilty of the charges and received varied jail sentences, while others got the death penalty.

23) **c:** Confidential information about a patient

Personal Identifying Information involves information about a patient. The loss of such personal and confidential information may cause the patient much embarrassment and inconvenience. Some of this information includes health-care insurance information and credit and debit card numbers.

24) **a:** It was created to address the issue of doctors who reportedly committed crimes during World War II

The Nuremberg Code was created to try medical doctors who committed atrocities against humanity during WWII.

25) **d:** Lawn mowers

Electrical equipment used in a medical facility includes ultrasound equipment, patient monitors and defibrillation pads. Although a hospital may have an electric lawn mower for the outside grounds, it is not a part of medical equipment.

26) **c:** Ease of exposure to hazardous substances and nature of their work

Safety symbols are a necessity in any workplace. They make the work environment safer and protect medical workers against infection.

27) **d:** All of the above

CT scans, ultrasounds and X-rays expose medical personnel to dangerous radiation.

28) **d:** All of the above

A fire in a hospital or a medical facility can lead to the destruction of property and medical equipment. It can also trigger panic and confusion. Loss of life is also another possibility.

29) **c:** History and Physical

History and Physical is an important reference document that contains valuable information, such as the patient's medical history and results of examinations done when the patient was admitted.

30) **c:** Both A and B

Aside from exposure to radiation, other accidents that medical workers in hospitals are prone to are work environment stress and falls or slips. Others are fire, laboratory hazards and exposure to infectious diseases through blood-borne pathogens.

31) **d:** A medical professional who specializes in treating ailments in the elderly

A geriatric medicine specialist focuses on ailments that are common to the elderly.

32) **b:** Coming into contact with patients' bodily fluids

There are several ways that medical workers are exposed to infections. While they sometimes may come in contact with radiation and droplets from sneezing and coughing, they most often are infected through contact with patients' bodily fluids.

33) **d:** No one should be exempted

Safety awareness has a purpose: to ensure that people are well informed about safety policies and procedures within a medical facility. Thus, when contemplating creating such awareness in a hospital, everyone must be involved, bar none.

34) **c:** Both A and B

Protective gear is recommended to protect medial workers against infections through contact with a patient's bodily fluids.

35) **a:** *Ante-* means in front of, while *ultra-* means beyond or excessive

Both *ultra-* and *ante-* are prefixes. However, they convey different meanings. *Ante-* means in front of or before, while *ultra-* means excessive or beyond. Examples are ultramodern and antenatal.

36) **b:** Bones, bone joints

Osseo- and *arthro-* are two prefixes with distinct meanings. The former is a prefix used for bones, while the latter is a prefix used for bone joints.

37) **d:** Two charts

Medical practitioners have access to two charts that assist them in using patients' medical records. These are Source-Oriented Medical Records and Problem-Oriented Medical Records.

38) **c:** *Rhino-*

The prefix *rhino-* is used for all medical terms that refer to the nose and nasal problems. Some examples of such medical terminology are rhinocele, rhinocephaly and rhinogenous.

39) **a:** A medical expert who specializes in treating eye diseases

An ophthalmologist is a medical expert whose area of specialization is treating eye diseases.

40) **b:** Endocrinologists

Endocrinologists treat a wide range of problems that include infertility, diabetes and thyroid problems. They specialize in treating hormones and metabolism issues.

41) **c:** Gastric bypass surgery

People who need to lose large quantities of weight can undergo gastric bypass surgery.

42) **b:** A medical condition characterized by hair loss or balding

Alopecia areata is a medical condition that affects hair follicles. Thus, it leads to hair loss and balding if not treated, because the damaged hair follicles prevent hair growth.

43) **d:** A group of diseases that cause painful blisters on the skin

A group of diseases that cause painful blisters on the skin is called epidermolysis bullosa. While the blisters are naturally painful, they become a real mess if they are infected.

44) **c:** Acute respiratory distress syndrome

As the name implies, this is a medical condition that is characterized by respiratory failure. Its symptoms include shortness of breath, rapid breathing and skin discoloration.

45) **a:** Problem-Oriented Medical Record

When at least two physicians are treating a medical problem simultaneously, the Problem-Oriented Medical Record is needed for the doctors to be on the same page. This is because it enables the physicians to document the illness and thus provides each doctor with the information needed to treat the ailment.

46) **c:** Mild traumatic brain injury

A mild traumatic brain injury is a medical condition that is triggered when someone is hit on the head repeatedly. It can also occur if an individual's head or body is shaken vigorously. The medical condition is commonly known as a concussion.

47) **a:** Plastic surgeon

A plastic surgeon is a medical professional who specializes in correcting major body anomalies through surgery. This medical expert can repair the skin or breasts or correct any deformity through surgical procedures.

48) **a:** If a patient will accept IV feeding or hydration as necessary

A patient may consider activating a living will under conditions such as whether he/she is willing to be tube-fed or receive IV hydration. It is also an option when considering whether to allow CPR or not.

49) **b:** The relationship between the prospective proxy candidate and the patient

A patient should consider several factors when choosing a proxy for the durable power of attorney. One such factor is the relationship between the patient and the prospective proxy. Delegating one's medical decisions to someone else is difficult. Trust is paramount.

50) **c:** A gynecologist or an obstetrician

A woman having difficulty conceiving or problems with her pregnancy should consult an obstetrician or a gynecologist.

51) **a:** State of residence

When considering whether to use a durable power of attorney, patients should factor in state of residence. This is because laws governing durable power of attorney differ from one state to another. Thus, a patient is advised to be familiar with the laws in his/her state.

52) **c:** Patients are not kept in the dark about their health

The objective of the Patient Self-Determination Act is to ensure that patients are fully informed during their treatment. They should be provided with all the information they need to make informed decisions. Thus, they should not be kept in the dark about their health.

53) **d:** Someone who has recently lost their home

Patients who are in a persistent vegetative state or who suffer from kidney disease or any severe mental condition may lose the power to make medical decisions. A stroke patient who is in a coma or who has cognitive deterioration loses that power as well.

54) **d:** It helps patients decide where to be treated

The Problem-Oriented Medical Record offers several benefits that include making documentation of chronic illnesses easier, assisting physicians when treating multiple illnesses simultaneously and helping patients be well informed about their condition. It does not empower patients to decide where to be treated.

55) **c:** A document written to discharge a patient from a hospital at the completion of treatment

The discharge summary is an important tool for medical physicians. This clinical report is usually prepared by a professional health-care provider at the completion of a patient's stay in the medical facility. It indicates that a patient is free to go home since the treatment has been completed.

56) **d:** A criminal offense

The Health Insurance Portability and Accountability Act was enacted as a part of an effort to regulate the medical profession. All physicians must comply with thc act. Failure to do so is considered a criminal offense under the law and incurs stiff penalties.

57) **b:** To prevent a threat to a patient's health or safety

Under the HIPAA Privacy Rule, health-care providers are permitted to disclose protected health information to prevent a threat to a patient's safety or health, if required by law enforcement agencies or if medical records are needed for government purposes.

58) **a:** Problem-Oriented Medical Record

The Problem-Oriented Medical Record is a method used in the medical field for recording important data about a patient's health status. This popular medical practice was introduced by Dr. Lawrence Weed in the 1950s.

59) **c:** It considers patients' responsibilities and rights when receiving medical care

The Patient Care Partnership addresses patients' responsibilities and rights when receiving medical care. It helps give patients a realistic view of their expectations and their own role in their medical treatment.

60) **d:** How patients can dictate the medical treatment they accept or reject

The Patient's Bill of Rights addresses some important issues, such as how patients can have access to the best medical care and how they can contribute to decisions involving their health. It also focuses on the importance of treating patients in a clean and safe environment.

61) **c:** It is a record of the patients in a medical facility

A medical record is a record of the patients in a medical facility. Each patient has a medical record where his/her personal information is kept. Both subjective data and objective data are recorded in each patient's medical record.

62) **d:** All of the above

A patient can be involved in his/her own medical care. Patients can decide the type of medical treatment they are comfortable with and also the type of treatment they will reject. When making decisions about their health, patients' opinions must be factored in. They must know the pros and cons of available treatment options.

63) **d:** Fundamental and Basic

The Source-Oriented Medical Record is divided into several subsections. Some of them are History and Physical, Diagnostic Testing and Nursing/Medical Assisting Notes. However, a SOMR does not have Fundamental and Basic subsections.

64) **d:** Informing the medical team of their financial status ahead of any medical treatment for billing purposes

A patient's responsibilities include telling health-care providers any pertinent important personal information that will assist doctors in providing treatment, notifying the medical team in advance prior to canceling an appointment and getting necessary information by asking relevant questions.

65) **d:** Consent to Treatment

Consent to Treatment is one of the most important rules guiding the medical professional and is fully supported by international human rights law. It specifically stipulates that someone must give express permission before the person is given any type of medical test, treatment or examination.

66) **d:** None of the above

Some branches of pediatrics are adolescent medicine, pediatric endocrinology and pediatric cardiology.

67) **c:** Source-Oriented Medical Record

SOMR means Source-Oriented Medical Record. It is a traditional data-recording format that is used for updating medical records. Some of its subdivisions are Progress Notes, History and Physical, and Diagnostic Testing.

68) **c:** Both A and B

Two conditions that must be satisfied for consent to treatment are that the consent must be given voluntarily, and the patient must understand the decision being made. Thus, a physician must provide adequate information that will enable patients to make informed decisions.

69) **b:** It is a medical condition with pimple-like bumps and boils as symptoms

Hidradenitis suppurativa is a non-contagious and chronic inflammatory health problem with boils or pimple-like bumps as symptoms. It can attack both beneath and above the skin. It is otherwise known as acne inversa.

70) **a:** Four

Four conditions must be met before a patient is considered to have the ability to make medical decisions. Patients must understand the information at their disposal, be able to retain the information, be able to process such information to make informed decisions and be able to communicate those decisions.

71) **b:** A flow sheet

A flow sheet is a document containing important data about a patient's condition. This document is usually kept in the patient's chart, where it can be referenced to provide information about the care given to the patient.

72) **b:** Written

Before a surgical procedure is carried out, the patient must express consent in writing. This waives any liability the medical team may have in case of any complications that may arise from the operation.

73) **d:** A document signed for a surgical procedure

This type of consent involves cooperating with the physician's instructions without expressing consent, either verbally or in writing. Examples of implied consent abound. Most times, you willingly submit to blood pressure tests, blood-sample taking and using medications.

74) **c:** Treating ailments common to infants through adolescents

Pediatrics are physicians who specialize in diagnosing and treating people from infancy through adolescence. Diseases common to infants such as allergies, asthma and croup are best handled by these experts.

75) **d:** All of the above

Some factors that influence some medical practitioners' attitudes toward their patients are poverty, prejudice, sexism and racism. Some patients may be given preferential treatment over others due to these factors.

76) **b:** The Hippocratic Allegiance and Regulatory Oath

Some of the regulations that all medical professionals are guided by are the Nuremberg Code, the Hippocratic Oath and the Declaration of Helsinki. The Hippocratic Allegiance and Regulatory Oath does not exist.

77) **a:** A source of ignition, a source of fuel and oxygen

Fire needs a source of ignition, a source of fuel and oxygen. In the absence of any of these, fire cannot exist.

78) **d:** Grounded power systems

To prevent electrical hazards, medical facilities should test their electrical devices on grounded power systems to identify shock risks and correct any problems.

79) **a:** Information about a patient sent to a doctor or received by a doctor

Clinical correspondence refers to information about a specific patient sent by a health organization or a doctor. It also refers to information received by a medical practitioner or an organization.

80) **b:** Rosacea

Rosacea is a long-term medical ailment that causes pimples and reddened skin. It mostly affects the face and can also trigger eye problems and thicken the skin.

81) **a:** Makes a list of work practices and grounding requirements for medical facilities

OSHA Standard 1910 established a list of grounding requirements and work practices that should be enforced in medical facilities to guarantee electrical safety in the workplace.

82) **d:** Reducing the number of health workers to prevent overcrowding

Accidents can be minimized in a medical facility if staff take precautions against blood-borne pathogens and are taught important safety policies. A compliance plan will also aid in compliance with established safety regulations. Reducing the number of health workers is never a solution to workplace safety.

83) **a:** Using protective equipment and reporting hazards immediately

Two components of the Safety and Health Management System are using protective equipment and reporting hazards immediately. The protective gear will shield you from possible exposure to harmful substances. Reporting hazards allows them to be corrected swiftly.

84) **a:** *Lacto-* is a prefix for milk, while *micro-* means small or tiny

Lacto- is a prefix for milk, while *micro-* means small or tiny.

85) **c:** A medical condition characterized by swelling and pain in the joints

This medical condition is known for causing pain and swelling in the joints. The condition usually arises when a tendon is repeatedly injured. The tendon is a part of the joint that is responsible for connecting the bones and muscles.

86) **d:** None of the above

All the words in the sentence are medical prefixes. You can visit the prefix section of this book for a list of medical prefixes, their meanings, usages and examples.

87) **d:** *Lapar-* and *pathologists*

Lapar- and *pathologists* are the odd words out of the given options. *-gnosis*, *-ecstasis* and *-itis* are suffixes. *Rhino-* is a prefix. Ophthalmologists and cardiologists are experts in different medical fields. However, *lapar-* is a prefix, while *pathologists* are medical professionals.

88) **a:** *Myo-*

Myo- is the prefix for describing medical terms for ailments that are associated with muscle tissue. Myoglobin, myocyte, myotonia and myocarditis are some examples of such words.

89) **c:** Immunologists

These professionals specialize in treating food allergies, asthma, insect sting allergies, eczema and other related immune system disorders. They are also referred to as allergists.

90) **c:** Specialists who treat issues with the nervous system

Neurologists focus primarily on treating issues relating to the nervous system and nerves. They treat diseases of the peripheral nerves, brain, autonomic nervous system, spinal cord and blood vessels. They also treat Alzheimer's disease, strokes and seizures.

91) **c:** Understand the connection between people's emotions and their mental health

Psychiatrists are medical experts who treat mental health. They are trained to understand the connection between people's emotions, their genetics and mental health.

92) **c:** Treat diseases affecting the internal organs

Internists are physicians who are primarily concerned with treating diseases affecting the internal organs. They treat diseases of the kidneys, heart, digestive system, joints, vascular system and respiratory system, irrespective of whether the diseases affect adults, adolescents or elderly patients.

93) **d:** Neurologists

The entire nervous system, including the spinal cord, the brain and the nerves, are specifically the domain of these medical specialists. People who suffer from Parkinson's disease, brain tumors, Alzheimer's disease and spinal tumors will be treated by neurologists.

94) **a:** It is a report about a patient written in his/her medical record after a surgical operation

It is a report about a patient written in his/her medical record after a surgical operation. In the note, the surgical procedure is documented to give insight into the entire process and provide information about the surgery to the medical staff.

95) **a:** POMR

POMR is helpful when treating a patient with complex medical conditions. Examples are patients with multimorbidity and other chronic ailments. Multiple clinicians must attend to their medical needs. These physicians' activities must be documented and coordinated to be effective.

96) **c:** Toward the left side of the midline

The heart is shaped like a closed fist and is roughly the same size as a man's closed fist. When seen through the midline, two-third of its entire mass, the larger part, is located toward the left side of the midline.

97) **a:** Excessive alcohol consumption and genetic diseases

Liver failure can be triggered by a wide range of factors that include genetic diseases and excessive alcohol consumption.

98) **b:** Internal and external organs

The female reproductive organs are divided into external and internal organs. The internal reproductive organs are the uterus, vagina, ovaries and fallopian tubes, while the external organs are the labia majora, clitoris and labia minora.

99) **a:** The shaft and the glans

The penis has two major parts, the glans and the shaft. The main penis part is the shaft, while the glans, otherwise called the head, is the tip. The glans has a small opening at its end for urination and ejaculation.

100) **d:** All of the above

When scheduling appointments, some factors you should take into consideration are late patients, patients' personal needs and physicians' preferences. Physician referrals, emergency calls and rescheduling canceled appointments are other factors that influence scheduling.

Practice Test 3

1. An effective way of ensuring that health-care providers keep up with their patients' needs is:
   a. Appointment scheduling
   b. Time analysis scheduling
   c. Time management analysis
   d. None of the above

2. Who is responsible for scheduling appointments?
   a. The medical team
   b. The physician
   c. The office assistant
   d. The medical assistant

3. Some of the factors to consider when scheduling appointments include:
   a. Physician and patient preferences
   b. Available facilities and physician preferences
   c. Duration of the visit and patient needs
   d. Physician preferences and duration of the examination

4. How many vital organs are in the body?
   a. Five
   b. Three
   c. Four
   d. Two

5. The primary function of the kidneys is:
   a. Blood circulation
   b. Blood production
   c. Blood filtration
   d. Blood distribution

6. What are basal ganglia?
    a. Parts of the brain responsible for movement coordination
    b. Parts of the nervous system responsible for coordinating the system
    c. Parts of the brain responsible for message coordination in the brain
    d. Parts of the brain specifically used for speech coordination

7. What is the primary function of the brainstem?:
    a. Controlling breathing and eating
    b. Controlling thoughts and emotions
    c. Controlling breathing and sleep
    d. Controlling breathing and digestion

8. What is the heart's primary function?
    a. Blood circulation throughout the body
    b. Blood circulation to only some important parts of the body
    c. Blood purification as a preventive measure against disease
    d. Supporting the circulatory system

9. Where are the lungs located?
    a. Below the abdominal sac
    b. On the right side of the chest
    c. On either side of the thorax
    d. Between the thorax and the chest

10. Why are two lobes located in the left lung?
    a. It is easier for them to function from the left lung than the right lung
    b. The left lung pumps more blood than the right lung
    c. The left lung is larger than the right lung
    d. The right lung does not have much power to power two lobes

11. Which of the following is not the metabolic function of the lungs?
    a. Synthesis of some substances
    b. Storage of some substances
    c. Degradation of some substances
    d. None of the above

12. Which of the following infectious agents have the ability to live in practically all types of environments?
    a. Bacteria
    b. Viruses
    c. Fungi
    d. Parasites

13. What is cirrhosis?
    a. A medical condition that affects the liver and leads to liver scarring
    b. A medical condition that affects the liver and leads to liver bloating
    c. A medical condition that affects the liver and leads to liver swelling
    d. A medical condition that affects the liver and leads to liver shrinking

14. What is the full meaning of COPD?
    a. Chronic organs pulmonary disease
    b. Chronic organ pulmonary disease
    c. Chronic obstructive pulmonary disease
    d. Chronic organs pulmonary disease

15. Define acute renal failure.
    a. A medical condition that leads to failure in the central nervous system
    b. A medical condition that leads to a malfunctioning respiratory system
    c. A medical condition that causes the kidneys to malfunction
    d. A medical condition that leads to chronic waist pain

16. Where does the body leave waste products?
    a. Bladder and kidneys
    b. Bowels and blood
    c. The kidneys and the two lungs
    d. The kidneys and the right lung

17. What is a measure taken by medical experts to prevent the spread of infection?
    a. Infection control and management
    b. Infection management and control
    c. Infection prevention and control
    d. Infection control

18. Which of the following is not a function of the kidneys?
    a. To balance bodily fluids
    b. To control some elements such as calcium and phosphorus
    c. To release the hormones the body needs for blood pressure control
    d. To serve as the channel between the bladder and the outside world

19. What is the bladder?
    a. A very important reproductive organ
    b. The main organ in the central nervous system
    c. A triangle-shaped organ that handles urine storage
    d. The urinary system organ that transports urine from one part of the body to the other before it is passed out as waste

20. What is droplet spread?
    a. The spread of infectious disease through urine
    b. The spread of infectious disease through blood
    c. The spread of infectious disease through kissing
    d. The spread of infectious disease through coughs and sneezes

21. Which is not performed by the reproductive system?
    a. Transporting cells
    b. Producing sperm cells and eggs
    c. Nurturing developing offspring
    d. Controlling waste product elimination

22. What functions do the fallopian tubes play?
    a. Sperm fertilization and allowing the fertilized eggs to move to the uterus' walls
    b. Sperm fertilization and segregation into female and male chromosomes
    c. Egg release and sperm development
    d. Sperm fertilization and development

23. Which of the following are not internal reproductive organs?
    a. Ovaries and fallopian tubes
    b. Vagina and uterus
    c. Fallopian tubes and uterus
    d. None of the above

24. The primary functions of the ovaries are:
    a. Producing, storing and releasing eggs into the fallopian tubes
    b. Producing urine, sperm and other bodily fluids
    c. Fertilizing sperm and eggs for pregnancy
    d. Making pregnancy smooth and easy

25. Diseases such as athlete's foot, impetigo and syphilis can be transferred through:
    a. Direct contact
    b. Indirect contact
    c. Droplet spread
    d. Sexual intercourse

26. What is the importance of penis stimulation during sexual intercourse?
    a. Stimulation hardens the penis and makes penetration easier
    b. It gives sperm enough strength to swim out of the penis
    c. Stimulation helps produce strong and healthy kids
    d. None of the above

27. What is incontinence?
    a. A medical condition common to the urinary system that causes urine leakage
    b. A medical condition that leads to colored urine and frequent urination
    c. A medical condition that is common to females of child-bearing age
    d. A medical condition common to female virgins

28. Define menstrual cramping.
    a. A menstrual problem characterized by thick menstrual flow
    b. A menstrual problem characterized by painful menstruation
    c. A menstrual problem with thick and painful menstruation
    d. A menstrual problem common to women approaching menopause

29. What is a type of cancer that affects the small gland that produces seminal fluid in males?
    a. Seminal fluid cancer
    b. Reproduction cancer
    c. Prostate cancer
    d. Prostatitis cancer

30. Erectile dysfunction can trigger some serious medical conditions, such as:
    a. Multiple sclerosis and trauma
    b. Some psychological issues and trauma
    c. Both A and B
    d. None of the above

31. What is a zygote made up of?
    a. 40 chromosomes; 20 from the egg and 20 from the sperm
    b. 40 chromosomes; 15 from the egg and 25 from the sperm
    c. 46 chromosomes; 20 from the egg and 26 from the sperm
    d. 46 chromosomes; 23 from the egg and 23 from the sperm

32. Which of the following is not a medium of virus transmission?
    a. Contaminated food or water
    b. Saliva exchanged during coughing or sneezing
    c. Transmission from insects or animals
    d. None of the above

33. What is a fomite?
    a. A medium through which infection transmission can be prevented
    b. An antiviral drug recommended for nursing mothers
    c. An inanimate object through which a virus can be transmitted
    d. An animate object through which a virus can be transmitted

34. What does the expression "parasites are microscopic" mean?
    a. It means that parasites transmit microscopic viruses to healthy people
    b. It means that parasites can hide under a microscope and escape being identified
    c. It means that parasites are so small they cannot be seen with the naked eye
    d. It means that some parasites are as big as a microscope

35. What are three examples of endemic fungi?
    a. Abdominal capsulatum, Histoplasma capsulatum and Immitis
    b. Immitis, Paracoccidioides brasiliensis and Blastomyces schenckii
    c. Sporothrix schenckii, Blastomyces dermatitidis and Coccidioides immitis
    d. None of the above

36. What are animal reservoirs?
    a. Giant pens built for keeping domestic animals
    b. Large enclosures built for keeping endangered species
    c. Animals that serve as infection transmission agents
    d. Animals that are used for researching potential antidotes to infectious diseases

37. What are two factors that determine a host's susceptibility to infection?
    a. Genetic factors and immunity
    b. Immunity and constitutional factors
    c. Both A and B
    d. None of the above

38. Handwashing as a preventive measure against infection is necessary under all of the following conditions except:
    a. When touching mucous membranes
    b. When touching medical equipment contaminated by bodily fluids
    c. After sneezing or coughing into a tissue
    d. After waking up in the morning

39. What does PPE protect against infection?
    a. Respiratory tract and skin
    b. Clothing and mucous membranes
    c. Both A and B
    d. None of the above

40. The effectiveness of most disinfectants is affected by several factors that include which of the following?
    a. Dirt and oil
    b. Oil and organic matter
    c. Organic matter and soap
    d. All washing liquids and solutions

41. What can data needed in a medical record can be divided into?
    a. Formative data and treatment data
    b. Admission data and informative data
    c. Subjective data and objective data
    d. Subjective data and formative data

42. During data collection, a medical worker's responsibilities include:
    a. Measuring physical attributes of a patient
    b. Recording findings and presenting the result to the physician in charge of the treatment
    c. Obtaining patients' medical history, social history and employment history
    d. All of the above

43. What is treatment compliance?
    a. The ability of a medical worker to abide by the rules and regulations guiding patient treatment
    b. A set of instructions a patient must be familiar with before being admitted to a medical facility
    c. The degree of a patient's willingness to obey medical directives
    d. A medical term for conditions guiding surgical procedures

44. According to some analyses, setting reminders can increase patients' treatment compliance rate by how much?
    a. 10%
    b. 12.76%
    c. 17.80%
    d. 27.95%

45. Who prepares patients for medical care?
    a. The senior physician
    b. The medical assistant
    c. Specialists specifically trained in patients' preparation
    d. Whoever is available to do the preparation

46. What are the two aspects of blood pressure that are considered?
    a. Systolic pressure and diastolic pressure
    b. Systolic pressure and demonstrative pressure
    c. Diastolic pressure and immune-derivate pressure
    d. Immune-derivate pressure and demonstrative pressure

47. A patient's pulse rate reads 150 beats per minute. Is the patient healthy or not?
    a. She is healthy
    b. She is not healthy
    c. Her health condition is a function of her state of mind
    d. Only a certified medical doctor can determine if she is healthy or not

48. What is one of the most effective ways to efficiently use resources?
    a. Through medical records
    b. Through regular resources review
    c. Through appointment scheduling
    d. Through interpersonal relationships with patients

49. Define wave scheduling.
    a. An appointment scheduling type that focuses on patient availability
    b. A method that involves planning a specific number of appointments within a specific period
    c. A method that involves planning a specific number of appointments over a long period of time
    d. An appointment scheduling type that focuses on health-care providers' availability

50. An appointment scheduling type that allows patients to see doctors according to their time of arrival is:
    a. Advanced scheduling
    b. Scheduled appointments
    c. Open office hours
    d. Flexible office hours

51. Which of the following is not a good appointment scheduling practice?
    a. Prioritizing some appointments
    b. Using appointment reminders
    c. Creating a waiting list
    d. Writing appointment dates on a calendar

52. Which factor should not be considered when scheduling appointments?
    a. Rescheduling canceled appointments
    b. Taking physician referrals into consideration
    c. Late patients
    d. Creating appointment logs for both new and old patients

53. What is a tickler file?
    a. A file organized to show the punctuality of each health worker
    b. A file containing necessary information about elderly patients
    c. A file with time-sensitive documents that health-care workers can use for scheduling time-based activities
    d. A collection of medical histories of new patients

54. What are nephrons?
    a. Nephrons are special nerves in the central nervous system that perform a wide range of functions
    b. Nephrons are tiny filters in the lungs that remove impurities and keep the lungs clean
    c. Nephrons are tiny filters in the intestines that remove impurities and keep the bowels clean
    d. Nephrons are tiny filters in the kidneys and support the kidneys to ensure that they function at maximum capacity

55. The human brain is:
    a. The most complex body part and a large body organ
    b. The most complex body part and the seat of motivation
    c. A simple body part that plays a very complex and sensitive role
    d. A simple body part with tens of thousands of nerves that perform an array of functions

56. What controls an individual's problem-solving abilities?
    a. Occipital lobes
    b. Temporal lobes
    c. Frontal lobes
    d. Adjacent lobes

57. What are two major functions of the liver?
    a. Filtering blood from the digestive tract and serving as a detoxification agent
    b. Filtering urine from the bladder and serving as a detoxification agent
    c. Filtering urine from the bladder and removing it through urination
    d. Supporting the secretion of sperm and sperm cells in the reproductive system

58. The heart's internal cavity is divided into the:
    a. Right atrium, left atrium, right ventricle and left ventricle
    b. Right atrium, left atrium, right ventrioles and left ventrioles
    c. Right electrum, left electrum, right ventricle and left ventricle
    d. Right atrium, left atrium, big ventricle and small ventricle

59. Air transportation through the tubular branches into the lungs is the primary function of the:
    a. Windpipe
    b. Right thorax
    c. Left bronchioles
    d. Air channel

60. How many lobes are in the right lung and how many lobes are in the left lung?
    a. Two and three
    b. Four and five
    c. Three and two
    d. One and two

61. Define hemochromatosis.
    a. A medical ailment triggered by the depositing of iron in the kidneys
    b. A medical ailment triggered by the depositing of iron in the liver
    c. A medical ailment triggered by the depositing of iron in the lower abdomen
    d. A medical ailment triggered by the depositing of iron in the left and right lungs

62. What is stable angina pectoris?
    a. A medical condition that is characterized by narrowed coronary arteries
    b. A medical condition that is characterized by elongated coronary arteries
    c. A medical condition that is characterized by expanded coronary arteries
    d. A medical condition that is characterized by inflamed coronary arteries

63. Define cardiomyopathy.
    a. An ailment that affects the heart muscle and changes its physical formation
    b. An ailment common to athletes that is characterized by painful muscle pull
    c. A medical condition that may lead to a lack of ability to engage in physical activities
    d. A medical condition that may result in swollen and painful legs

64. Define congestive heart failure.
    a. Failure of the heart resulting from prolonged use under certain conditions
    b. Heart failure caused by overexposure to carcinogenic substances
    c. Heart failure triggered by a severe, untreated heart problem
    d. A heart problem with sneezing, coughing and sweating as symptoms

65. Which of the following ailments is caused by an abnormal inflammation of the lungs' airways?
    a. Pleurisy
    b. Asthma
    c. Bronchiectasis
    d. Chronic obstructive pulmonary disease

66. What is a symptom of cystic fibrosis?
    a. Inability to stand erect due to pain in the legs and back
    b. Difficulty in holding urine, leading to urine leakage
    c. Difficulty in expelling mucus from the airway easily
    d. Difficulty in passing waste products from the body

67. Which of the following ailments are kidney problems?
    a. Acute renal failure and nephrotic syndrome
    b. Pyelonephritis and nephrotic syndrome
    c. Nephrogenic diabetes insipidus and papillary necrosis
    d. All of the above

68. What is the body system?
    a. A group of systems controlling the body's metabolism
    b. A group of systems controlling the body's central nervous system
    c. A group of systems controlling the body's respiratory system
    d. A group of systems controlling the body's functions

69. Which body releases the hormone needed for controlling the amount and volume of red blood cells produced in the body?
    a. The kidneys
    b. The left and right centrioles
    c. The middle and left lungs
    d. The respiratory system

70. What is the function of the nerves in the bladder?
    a. They ensure the filtration of urine in the bladder
    b. They regulate the amount of urine the bladder can hold
    c. They clean the bladder and ensure it is free from any infection caused by the urine
    d. They alert people of the need to empty the bladder when necessary

71. Which is not a function of the reproductive system?
    a. Egg and sperm cell production
    b. Hormone production
    c. Transportation of produced cells
    d. Egg division into nuclei

72. How does the reproductive system get rid of unfertilized eggs?
    a. Through fetal removal
    b. Through wet dreams
    c. Through menstruation
    d. Through a surgical procedure

73. How is the vagina kept moist and protected?
    a. By washing with water and soap regularly
    b. By applying lubrication twice daily
    c. Through the mucous membranes in its muscular walls
    d. Through some special medical procedures

74. Which female organ has the strongest muscles that can expand and contract?
    a. The vagina
    b. The uterus
    c. The fallopian tubes
    d. The reproductive organs

75. What are the female reproductive system's two external organs?
    a. Small and large labia
    b. Labia majora and labia minora
    c. Left labia and right labia
    d. Reproductive labia and respiratory labia

76. What are the male reproductive organs?
    a. The duct system and the accessory glands
    b. The penis and the duct system
    c. The testicles and the penis
    d. All of the above

77. What reproductive transformation does a male experience at puberty?
    a. Some hormones and testosterone trigger the transformation of cells into sperm cells
    b. Some hormones and testosterone trigger the transformation of multidimensional cells into sperm cells
    c. Some hormones and testosterone trigger the transformation of complex cells into sperm cells
    d. Some hormones and testosterone trigger the transformation of simple cells into sperm cells

78. What are the components of semen?
    a. Sperm and water
    b. Sperm and blood
    c. Seminal fluid and sperm
    d. Penis discharge and seminal fluid

79. What is interstitial cystitis otherwise known as?
    a. Chronic bladder infectious disease
    b. Bladder swelling and inflammation
    c. Painful bladder syndrome
    d. None of the above

80. Define endometriosis.
    a. A medical condition that affects the endometrium
    b. A medical condition that affects the endometric palate
    c. A medical condition that affects the endometrium biopsis
    d. A medical condition that affects the endometrium congenital labia

81. Which of the following is not a component of a virus?
    a. Deoxyribonucleic acid
    b. Ribonucleic acid
    c. A coat of protein or lipid
    d. A protective shell that increases viral resistance to drugs

82. What are parasites?
    a. Carriers of infection from inanimate objects and animals to humans
    b. Living organisms that depend on other living organisms for existence
    c. Drug-resistant infection carriers common in arid regions
    d. Microscopic infection carriers common in cold regions

83. Which of these pairs of infection carriers are not parasites?
    a. Stomach worms and protozoa
    b. Skin mites and crab lice
    c. Hookworm and giardiasis
    d. Ebola and rabies

84. What is dimorphic yeast?
    a. Multifunctional yeast
    b. A special form of yeast that can withstand any type of environment
    c. An infectious disease from the yeast family
    d. A common form of bacteria that transmits disease from one person to another

85. People come in direct contact with some infectious diseases through which of the following?
    a. Sharing personal effects
    b. Hugging and shaking hands
    c. Both A and B
    d. None of the above

86. The following are two major factors that affect vector-borne diseases:
    a. Temperature and rainfall
    b. Rainfall and snow
    c. Temperature and atmospheric conditions
    d. Existing climatic condition and individuals' immunity to disease

87. Oral transmission refers to which of the following?
    a. The accidental consumption of foods that can lower one's sexual prowess
    b. The accidental consumption of contaminated food or water
    c. Swallowing oral medication
    d. None of the above

88. An infectious disease cannot survive in the absence of which of the following?
    a. Water, air and food
    b. Light, water and air
    c. A host, an agent and an environment
    d. All of the above

89. What is a portal of exit?
    a. The point where waste products are discharged from the body
    b. A mechanism for treating some terminal diseases
    c. The channel through which a transmission agent leaves the host's body
    d. The point of death for a terminal ailment

90. Which of the following is an effective preventive measure against infectious diseases?
    a. Proper nose hygiene
    b. Proper hand hygiene
    c. Proper home maintenance
    d. Proper mouth and nose hygiene

91. What's the best way to handle used PPE?
    a. Wash it with water and soap for 48 hours
    b. Wash it with an alcohol-based solution for 24 hours
    c. Dispose of it immediately
    d. Wash it with a combination of soap, water and alcohol-based solution and dry clean

92. Which of the following are the recommended disinfectants for medical facilities?
    a. EPA-registered disinfectants
    b. EPA-registered and NPA-regulated disinfectants
    c. NPA-registered and EPA-regulated disinfectants
    d. Specially formulated disinfectants for specific uses

93. Sharp objects are best disposed of in:
    a. Leak-proof and transparent containers
    b. Puncture-resistant and leak-proof containers
    c. Big and cold containers
    d. Tough and red-colored containers

94. Disposable rags, cloths and used PPE are best disposed of in which of the following?
    a. Leak-proof and transparent containers
    b. Biohazard containers
    c. Big and cold containers
    d. Fragile containers

95. Differentiate between subjective data and objective data.
    a. Subjective data are obtained from the public medical database, while objective data are provided by patients themselves
    b. Objective data are obtained from the public medical database, while objective data are provided by patients themselves
    c. Subjective data are provided by patients themselves, while objective data are obtained by the medical team through tests and diagnostics
    d. Objective data are provided by patients themselves, while subjective data are obtained by the medical team through tests and diagnostics

96. Some examples of objective data are:
    a. General appearance and body temperature
    b. Symptoms of morning sickness and general appearance
    c. Body temperature and loss of appetite
    d. None of the above

97. Which of the following is a helpful tip to encourage patient compliance?
    a. Public service campaigns
    b. Reminding patients regularly
    c. Educating patients
    d. All of the above

98. What factors affect treatment compliance?
    a. Complexity of treatment and patients' lack of knowledge about their sickness
    b. Patients' socioeconomic status and weight
    c. Lack of adequate medical facilities to enforce treatment compliance
    d. Lack of support from the government and absence of durable power of attorney

99. Which of the following is a first step toward patient preparation?
    a. Creating awareness about the potential side effects of a given treatment
    b. Preparing the treatment room in advance
    c. Setting a reminder for the treatment
    d. Obtaining written permission from the patient before the treatment commences

100. The normal respiration rate for a healthy adult is:
    a. Between 15 and 20 breaths per minute
    b. Between 20 and 30 breaths per minute
    c. Between 10 and 20 breaths per minute
    d. Between 12 and 16 breaths per minute

Practice Test 3 – Answers

1) **a:** Appointment scheduling

Appointment scheduling is an effective means of ensuring that health-care providers keep up with the demand for their attention, especially when a huge number of their patients need their attention within the same time frame.

2) **d:** The medical assistant

When a physician is overwhelmed with work, it is your responsibility as a medical assistant to schedule appointments. Thus, you determine who visits the physician, when and for how long.

3) **b:** Available facilities and physician preferences

Available facilities and physician preferences are two of the factors that a medical assistant should consider when scheduling appointments. These factors take into consideration the need to ensure that the right facilities are used for medical procedures as well as ensuring appointments are scheduled at convenient times for the physician.

4) **a:** Five

There are five vital organs in the body. These are the kidneys, liver, lungs, brain and heart.

5) **c:** Blood filtration

The kidneys are designed to filter blood. During filtration, they ensure that the body's fluids are balanced in addition to removing waste. They also keep the body's electrolytes at the right levels.

6) **c:** Parts of the brain responsible for message coordination in the brain

In the center of the brain is a cluster of structures that form the basal ganglia. It is responsible for coordinating messages between several other brain parts and areas of the body.

7) **c:** Controlling breathing and sleep

This part of the brain is responsible for controlling some basic functions, such as sleep and breathing.

8) **a:** Blood circulation throughout the body
In the human body, the circulatory system revolves around the heart. The four-chambered double pump is between the two lungs, where they ensure that the body receives the needed amount of blood for proper functioning.

9) **c:** On either side of the thorax

The lungs are located on either side of the thorax. They are spongy and filled with air. They are also soft and elastic. At birth, both lungs contain some air. Healthy lungs float in water, and when squeezed, they will crackle.

10) **c:** The left lung is larger than the right lung

Each lung is divided into lobes. A tissue fissure separates the lobes from one another. There are three lobes in the right lung. The left lung has two lobes because it is bigger than the right lung.

11) **d:** None of the above

The lungs support metabolism. Through their metabolic functions, they are able to support the synthesis of some substances, store some substances and also degrade some substances when necessary.

12) **b:** Viruses

Viruses are infectious agents with the ability to live in a wide range of environments.

13) **a:** A medical condition that affects the liver and leads to liver scarring

Cirrhosis is a medical condition that arises when the liver is damaged. The permanent damage may cause the liver to be scarred for good.

14) **c:** Chronic obstructive pulmonary disease

COPD means chronic obstructive pulmonary disease. It is a health problem that may be triggered by cigarette smoking, genetic conditions, infectious diseases and air pollution. When the lungs are damaged, they find it increasingly difficult to function at maximum capacity. This may cause breathing difficulties.

15) **c:** A medical condition that causes the kidneys to malfunction

This medical condition is characterized by a sudden depreciation in the kidneys' functioning power. Several causes may include kidney damage or a blockage of the urinary tract. It is also referred to as kidney failure.

16) **b:** Bowels and blood

The body leaves waste products in the blood and bowel before they are eventually removed in either solid or liquid form through urination and bowel emptying.

17) **d:** Infection control

Infection control is implemented to prevent infection from spreading across communities, among patients and medical staff, and within health-care facilities.

18) **d:** To serve as the channel between the bladder and the outside world

The kidneys balance the body's fluids, release the hormones the body needs for blood pressure control and control some elements in the body such as phosphorus and calcium.

19) **c:** It is a triangle-shaped organ that handles urine storage

The bladder is a hollow organ in the lower belly. The triangle-shaped organ stores urine due to the expansion and relaxation of its walls. A healthy adult can store about two cups of urine for up to five hours.

20) **d:** The spread of infectious disease through coughs and sneezes

When someone sneezes or coughs, he/she may spray droplets of saliva. These droplets may transmit an infection to a healthy person who comes in contact with them. People at a close distance may also be infected.

21) **d:** Controlling waste product elimination

Some of the functions that the reproductive system performs are sperm cell and egg production, transporting the produced cells and nurturing developing offspring. Waste product elimination is not a function of the reproductive system.

22) **a:** Sperm fertilization and allowing the fertilized eggs to move to the uterus' walls

The fallopian tubes are narrow tubes attached to the uterus' upper part. They transport ova to the uterus from the ovaries. Fertilization occurs in the fallopian tubes. After fertilization, eggs move to the uterus, where they are implanted into the uterine wall lining.

23) **d:** None of the above

The female reproductive system is divided into internal and external reproductive organs. The internal organs are made up of the vagina, the uterus, ovaries and fallopian tubes.

24) **a:** Producing, storing and releasing eggs into the fallopian tubes

The ovaries are a part of the internal reproductive organs. They produce eggs in the reproductive system, store the eggs and eventually release them into the fallopian tubes.

25) **a:** Direct contact

Diseases can be transferred in a couple of ways. Diseases such as athlete's foot, syphilis and impetigo are transmitted through direct contact with a carrier.

26) **a:** Stimulation hardens the penis and makes penetration easier

During sexual intercourse, a hard penis can easily penetrate the vagina.

27) **a:** A medical condition common to the urinary system that causes urine leakage

Victims of this ailment usually have the urge to urinate frequently; urine leakage is another common symptom, especially in women.

28) **b:** A menstrual problem characterized by painful menstruation

Menstrual cramps are a severe problem associated with the female monthly menstrual flow. It is the most common female reproductive system medical condition. It is medically known as dysmenorrhea.

29) **c:** Prostate cancer

Prostate cancer is a medical condition of the male reproductive system. It affects the small gland that produces the seminal fluid used for nourishing and transporting sperm. It is the most common disease that affects the male reproductive organs and can result in medical conditions such as frequent urination and erectile dysfunction.

30) **c:** Both A and B

Erectile dysfunction is a medical condition in which a man cannot get an erection or is unable to sustain an erection for sexual intercourse. The medical condition can also trigger vascular disease and a host of neurological disorders such as trauma, multiple sclerosis and some psychological issues.

31) **d:** 46 chromosomes; 23 from the egg and 23 from the sperm

A fertilized egg is known as a zygote. It is made up of 46 chromosomes, 23 chromosomes from the sperm and the other half from the egg. Then, both combine to form a new individual.

32) **d:** None of the above

Viruses can be transmitted from one individual to another in a number of ways. Some mediums of virus transmission are through contaminated food or water, saliva exchange during sneezing or coughing and via animals and insects.

33) **c:** An inanimate object through which a virus can be transmitted

Fomites are inanimate objects that serve as a means of transmitting infections from an infected person to a healthy person. Elevator buttons, doorknobs, phones, handrails, keyboards and a host of other objects that many people share regularly are common examples of fomites.

34) **c:** It means that parasites are so small that they cannot be seen with the naked eye

A microscopic organism is an organism that is so small that it cannot be seen without the assistance of magnifying objects such as a microscope. Thus, parasites are so small that the naked eyes cannot see them unaided.

35) **c:** Sporothrix schenckii, Blastomyces dermatitidis and Coccidioides immitis

Dimorphic yeast can live in humans and a wide range of environments where it can transfer evasive diseases that otherwise healthy humans are not immune to. Some examples are Blastomyces dermatitidis, Histoplasma capsulatum, Sporothrix schenckii, Coccidioides immitis and Paracoccidioides brasiliensis. These agents are otherwise known as endemic fungi.

36) **c:** Animals that serve as infection transmission agents

Some animals transmit infections from one person to another. Some of the diseases such animals transmit are anthrax, brucellosis, tularemia, monkeypox and rabies. Such animals are known as animal reservoirs.

37) **c:** Both A and B

Some factors that determine the degree to which a host is susceptible to infection include immunity and genetics. A host's resistance to infection may be increased or decreased by individual genetics.

38) **d:** After waking up in the morning

Handwashing is a very effective infection-prevention practice. People at risk of infection should wash their hands after sneezing or coughing into a tissue, when touching medical equipment contaminated by bodily fluids and when touching mucous membranes. Washing your hands when you wake up in the morning is needless.

39) **a:** Respiratory tract and skin

Personal protective equipment protects the respiratory tract, clothing, skin and mucous membranes against infection. The equipment includes protective items, such as masks, gloves, respirators, gowns and eyewear.

40) **b:** Oil and organic matter

The effectiveness of most disinfectants is affected by several factors that include oil and organic matter. This explains why it is important that surfaces such as walls and floors are clean before disinfecting them.

41) **c:** Subjective data and objective data

The data needed in a medical record can be divided into objective data and subjective data. While objective data refers to the physical data that you can personally observe, subjective data refers to the information provided by a patient.

42) **d:** All of the above

During data collection, a medical worker's responsibilities include measuring physical attributes of a patient, obtaining a patient's social and medical history, recording findings and presenting the results to the appropriate physician.

43) **c:** The degree of a patient's willingness to obey medical directives

Treatment compliance refers to the degree to which a patient is willing to abide by medical directives, attend appointments, follow medical regimens and engage in preventive care as recommended by the patient's health-care provider.

44) **c:** 17.80%

Some patients who struggle with keeping medical appointments or with following through on treatment may need reminders. According to some research, such reminders may improve adherence rates by 17.8%.

45) **b:** The medical assistant

A medical assistant is responsible for prepping patients for medical care. Other responsibilities include updating medical records, assisting with scheduling appointments, assisting physicians with diagnosis, preparing laboratory samples and preparing patients for examinations.

46) **a:** Systolic pressure and diastolic pressure

When reading blood pressure, the systolic pressure and diastolic pressure are taken into consideration. This refers to the measurement taken after the contraction of the heart and before the contraction respectively. The higher figure represents the systolic pressure, while the lower figure represents the diastolic pressure.

47) **b:** She is not healthy

If a patient's pulse reads 150 beats per minute, the patient is unhealthy. This is because the pulse rate for a healthy adult is between 60 and 120 beats per minute.

48) **c:** Through appointment scheduling

Appointment scheduling is an effective means of managing and utilizing resources efficiently. With well-planned appointments, physicians will not waste time waiting for a patient while there are other patients to be attended to. That saves time and other resources, increasing the physician's efficiency.

49) **b:** A method that involves planning a specific number of appointments within a specific period

Wave scheduling offers some flexibility. It involves planning a specific number of appointments within a specific period of time. Thus, the appointments are attended to on a first-come, first-served basis. Whoever misses their appointment loses that opportunity until another time.

50) **c:** Open office hours

Patients are allowed to see the doctor in order of their arrival. This completely eliminates appointment cancelation or situations in which some patients arrive for their appointments far behind schedule. It is the most popular appointment type and is practiced by all medical facilities by default.

51) **d:** Writing appointment dates on a calendar

A well-planned appointment schedule can help keep doctors from being overwhelmed. Some valuable tips when scheduling appointments include prioritizing appointments, using appointment reminders and creating a waiting list. These are better tools than a calendar.

52) **d:** Creating appointment logs for both new and old patients

When scheduling appointments, consider that some patients are habitually late to appointments, some canceled appointments may be rescheduled, and a physician may receive referrals from colleagues. Creating appointment logs for both new and old patients is not a factor.

53) **c:** A file with time-sensitive documents that health-care workers can use for scheduling time-based activities

A ticker file is otherwise known as a 43 Folder System. It is a collection of file folders with some specific days. The file is organized so that time-sensitive documents can easily be retrieved for use.

54) **d:** Nephrons are tiny filters in the kidneys and support the kidneys to ensure that they function at maximum capacity

Each kidney has about one million nephrons. These are tiny filters that support the kidneys' functions and ensure that they are healthy and function at maximum capacity.

55)**a:** The most complex body part and a large body organ

The human brain is undoubtedly the most complex body part aside from ranking among the largest body organs. The brain is the control center of the entire body.

56) **c:** Frontal lobes

The human brain consists of many lobes, such as the parietal lobe, frontal lobes, temporal lobes and occipital lobes, all performing distinct functions in the brain. An individual's problem-solving abilities are controlled by the frontal lobes. They are also responsible for people's motor function and judgment.

57) **a:** Filtering blood from the digestive tract and serving as a detoxification agent

The liver is one of the five vital body organs. As an important body part, it serves as a detoxification agent and filters blood from the digestive tract. In these capacities, it removes impurities from the blood and removes toxins from the body.

58) **a:** Right atrium, left atrium, right ventricle and left ventricle

The heart's internal cavity is divided into four layers. These are the right atrium, the left atrium, the right ventricle and the left ventricle. Each layer contributes to the overall function and performance of the heart.

59) **a:** Windpipe

The windpipe inhales air through the bronchi, or tubular branches, into the lungs. Then, the tubular branches divide into bronchioles until they become microscopic. Another name for the windpipe is trachea.

60) **c:** Three and two

There are three lobes in the right lung. The left lung has two lobes because it is bigger than the right lung. The asymmetrical shape of the heart is responsible for the differences in sizes of the pair of lungs.

61) **b:** A medical ailment triggered by the depositing of iron in the liver

This ailment is triggered by the depositing of iron in the liver. The deposited iron damages the liver gradually. Iron is also deposited in other parts of the body, causing multiple health problems.

62) **a:** A medical condition that is characterized by narrowed coronary arteries

When the coronary arteries are narrowed, this can result in discomfort or chest pain. As a result of the blockage, the heart is denied the extra oxygen it needs to carry out strenuous activities. That can have a huge negative impact on the heart.

63) **a:** An ailment that affects the heart muscle and changes its physical formation

This ailment affects the heart muscle. The muscle becomes abnormally thick, enlarged or stiff. This is in addition to other physical changes. When the heart's physical shape is altered, its efficiency is negatively affected.

64) **c:** Heart failure triggered by a severe, untreated heart problem

The heart has four valves. When any of the valves develops a problem, congestive heart failure may result.

65) **c:** Bronchiectasis

An abnormal inflammation of the lungs' airways is the primary cause of bronchiectasis. It may also arise from the impact on the bronchi. Either condition may cause bronchiectasis, especially after the lung has been subjected to repeated infections. The ailment's main symptom is repeated coughing.

66) **c:** Difficulty in expelling mucus from the airway easily

Cystic fibrosis is a genetic condition that is characterized by difficulty in expelling from mucus the airway easily. The excess mucus that cannot be easily cleared leads to repeated cases of pneumonia and bronchitis.

67) **d:** All of the above

Acute renal failure, pyelonephritis, nephrotic syndrome, nephrogenic diabetes insipidus and papillary necrosis are some common kidney problems. If not properly or promptly treated, the heart may malfunction or fail completely.

68) **d:** A group of systems controlling the body's functions

The body system is a group of systems controlling the body's functions. Some of the major systems are the respiratory system, urinary system, reproductive system and central nervous system.

69) **a:** The kidneys

The kidneys release the hormones needed to control the amount and volume of red blood cells produced by the body. They also release hormones that are needed to control blood pressure.

70) **d:** They alert people of the need to empty the bladder when necessary

The nerves send signals to people to empty their bladder when it is full of urine.

71) **d:** Egg division into nuclei

The reproductive system is solely concerned with reproduction. It produces egg cells, sperm cells and hormones and transports the produced cells to the right part of the body.

72) **c:** Through menstruation

Sperm from a male fertilizes the eggs produced in the female reproductive system. However, if the eggs are not fertilized, the female will expel the unfertilized eggs through menstruation.

73) **c:** Through the mucous membranes in its muscular walls

The body has a natural way of protecting the vagina and keeping it moist. Its muscular walls are lined with mucous membranes for that purpose.

74) **b:** The uterus

The uterus is commonly known as the womb. It has muscular walls and a thick lining. The muscles are stronger than most muscles in any female and can contract and expand, allowing a growing fetus enough space to grow. The muscles are also used for pushing a baby out during childbirth.

75) **b:** Labia majora and labia minora

The external organs of the female reproductive system are the labia majora and labia minora. The former are the bigger of the two and protect the external reproductive organs by enclosing them, while the latter are located inside the majora and surround the urethra.

76) **d:** All of the above

The male reproductive organs are the duct system, accessory glands, testicles and penis. Within the reproductive context, they are used for sperm and egg production, coitus and the release of sperm into the vagina to fertilize eggs in the fallopian tubes.

77) **d:** Some hormones and testosterone trigger the transformation of simple cells into sperm cells

When a male reaches puberty, testosterone and other hormones trigger the transformation of simple cells in the tubules into sperm cells. The cells undergo division and transformation until each assumes a tadpole-like structure with a short tail and head. Safely kept in the head is genetic material.

78) **c:** Seminal fluid and sperm

During sexual stimulation of a male, the seminal fluid will form semen by mixing with sperm. The stimulation also leads to the hardening of the once limp penis, a sign of sexual excitement. The tissues in the penis will subsequently be filled with blood that makes it erect and stiff.

79) **c:** Painful bladder syndrome

Another name for this ailment that is common to the urinary system is painful bladder syndrome. Chronic bladder problems are common in women. Pelvic pain is another common syndrome.

80) **a:** A medical condition that affects the endometrium

This medical condition affects the endometrium, the inside of the uterus. It gradually moves to the outside of the uterus and affects organs such as the bowels, ovaries and the tissue lining the victim's pelvis. When the endometrial tissue is trapped, it results in a painful medical condition.

81) **d:** A protective shell that increases viral resistance to drugs

Viruses are made up of DNA or RNA. They are usually surrounded by a coat of lipids, proteins or glycoproteins, proof of their complexity. They are parasitic organisms and thrive only in the presence of a host.

82) **b:** Living organisms that depend on other living organisms for existence

Parasites are living organisms whose existence depends on another living organism. They are mostly disease carriers and may undermine their host's health. Some parasites gain entrance to the host's body through contaminated water or food, while some live on the host's hair or skin.

83) **d:** Ebola and rabies

They are mostly disease carriers and may undermine their host's health. Some examples of parasites are protozoa, stomach worms, skin mites, crab lice, giardiasis and hookworm. Ebola and rabies are not parasites.

84) **b:** A special form of yeast that can withstand any type of environment

Dimorphic yeast is a special fungus that can survive in any environment. This makes it easier to transfer diseases from one person to another across a wide range of environments.

85) **c:** Both A and B

People can come in direct contact with infectious diseases while sharing personal effects such as towels, socks and other clothing, especially if such items are not thoroughly washed before they are shared with others. Direct contact also includes hugging and shaking hands.

86) **a:** Temperature and rainfall

Vector-borne diseases are the leading causes of mortality and morbidity in the world, although subtropical and tropical countries are hit hardest by such devastating diseases. The major factors that affect vector-borne diseases are rainfall and temperature.

87) **b:** The accidental consumption of contaminated food or water

Oral transmission occurs when a healthy person accidentally consumes contaminated water or food, leading to the ingestion of harmful organisms. Chewing or licking contaminated surfaces or objects can result in ingestion, too. Feces, exudate, saliva or urine may contaminate an object through which the pathogenic organism may be ingested.

88) **c:** A host, an agent and an environment

An infectious disease needs six elements to survive: a host, an agent, an environment, a portal of exit, a portal of entry and a reservoir. These elements combine to form the chain of infection. The absence of any of the members of the chain signals the death of an infectious disease.

89) **c:** The channel through which a transmission agent leaves the host's body

A portal of exit refers to the channel through which a transmission agent leaves the host's body. The location of the pathogen, more often than not, corresponds to the portal of exit. For instance, Mycobacterium tuberculosis affects the respiratory tract, and that serves as its portal of exit as well.

90) **b:** Proper hand hygiene

Proper hand hygiene is an effective preventive measure against infectious diseases. Washing your hands regularly with soap and water will reduce your vulnerability to infections. Alternatively, you may keep your hands clean with alcohol-based sanitizers.

91) **c:** Dispose of it immediately

Personal protection equipment is equipment that medical workers may wear to protect themselves against infection. PPE includes a face mask, goggles and a gown. After using PPE, it should be disposed of in the appropriate trash can immediately.

92) **a:** EPA-registered disinfectants

EPA-registered disinfectants are recommended for medical facilities. They contain manufacturers' instructions with information on the amount of disinfectant to use and the dilution ratio.

93) **b:** Puncture-resistant and leak-proof containers

The best way to dispose of sharp objects is to dispose of them in puncture-resistant and leak-proof containers. Such containers are sturdy and durable. They will not be easily damaged by the sharp objects.

94) **b:** Biohazard containers

Biohazard containers are best for disposing of disposable rags, PPE and cloths. Such bags should not be easily breakable or punctured. Ensure that you use a leak-proof bag with the appropriate biohazard symbol for easy identification.

95) **c:** Subjective data are provided by patients themselves, while objective data are obtained by the medical team through tests and diagnostics

Physicians need two types of data from a patient for diagnosis and treatment: subjective data and objective data. Subjective data are provided by patients themselves, while objective data are obtained by the medical team through tests and diagnosis.

96) **d:** None of the above

A physician can personally see objective data. Heart rate, weight, blood pressure, height, general appearance and body temperature are examples of objective data. General appearance, symptoms of any ailment and loss of appetite are not objective data.

97) **d:** All of the above

Patient compliance can be encouraged by creating public service campaigns that highlight the importance of compliance, supporting patients regularly and educating patients about the consequences of not complying with medical advice.

98) **a:** Complexity of treatment and patients' lack of knowledge about their sickness

Patient ignorance is influenced by several factors. Two such factors are lack of knowledge about the sickness and complexity of the treatment. Others are inadequate follow-up, cognitive impairment, psychological problems and medication side effects.

99) **b:** Preparing the treatment room in advance

When preparing a patient for any medical procedure, the first step is to ensure that the treatment room is in order before the treatment commences. This involves keeping the room clean as well as ensuring that all needed tools and equipment are prepared.

100) **d:** Between 12 and 16 breaths per minute

The respiration rate of an individual is the number of breaths a person takes per minute. It is typically calculated by counting the number of times a person's chest rises. A healthy adult has a normal respiration range of between 12 and 16 breaths per minute.

Practice Test 4

1. How many vital signs are in the human body?
    a. Five
    b. Six
    c. Eight
    d. Four

2. What is the range of the human body temperature?
    a. 36°C and 37.2°C
    b. 36.5°C and 37.2°C
    c. 36.5°C and 37°C
    d. 36.5°C and 47.2°C

3. Which of the following are benefits of treatment compliance?
    a. It is cost-effective and improves health
    b. It improves health
    c. It is effective and easy to practice
    d. It is relatively easy to implement

4. When conducting a physical examination on a patient, a medical professional should measure which of the following?
    a. Weight and height
    b. Social status and financial status
    c. Hand reach and ability to withstand pain
    d. None of the above

5. Which are not examples of subjective data?
    a. Exhaustion and itching
    b. Shortness of breath and pain
    c. Dizziness and coughing
    d. None of the above

6. Which are not examples of objective data?
    a. Blood pressure and heart rate
    b. General appearance and body temperature
    c. Height and weight
    d. Vomiting and dizziness

7. What information does a health worker collect first when collecting subjective data?
    a. The patient's present ailment
    b. The patient's major complaint
    c. The patient's medical history
    d. The patient's family medical history

8. Asking what ailment the patient has been treated for recently gives insight into the patient's:
    a. Present ailment
    b. Past medical history
    c. Social history
    d. Medical record

9. Which of the following are examples of fomites?
    a. Toilets and doorknobs
    b. Sinks and rails
    c. Door handles and bus seats
    d. All of the above

10. When are surgical masks and goggles best worn?
    a. When a medical worker is at high risk of being contaminated by bodily fluids
    b. When they are readily available
    c. When there is a surplus supply of protective gear
    d. When performing any medical procedure

11. Which of the following is the best way to disinfect soiled hands?
    a. Water and soap
    b. An alcohol-based solution
    c. A solution of water and any disinfectant
    d. A solution of soap and any cleaning agent

12. It appropriate to wash your hands in all of the following situations except:
    a. When you touch a contaminated object with bare hands
    b. When you touch a contaminated object even if you wear gloves
    c. When you feel it is necessary to do so
    d. When you feel some symptoms of infection

13. Which is a factor that determines a host's resistance to infection?
    a. Genetic makeup
    b. Social and financial status
    c. Degree of exposure to infection
    d. Natural ability to get over infection without medical assistance

14. The final link in the chain of infection is:
    a. The environment
    b. A new host
    c. The reservoir
    d. None of the above

15. What is the portal of entry?
    a. The channel through which a transmission agent leaves the host's body
    b. The channel through which a transmission agent enters the host's body
    c. The stage at which the infection can be effectively controlled
    d. The stage at which an infection is beyond control

16. Ingestion can take place through food or objects contaminated with:
    a. Saliva and urine
    b. Blood and urine
    c. Sputum and tears
    d. All of the above

17. Yellow fever is which of the following?
    a. A vector-borne disease transmitted by rodents
    b. A vector-borne disease transmitted by animals and birds
    c. A vector-borne disease transmitted by the anopheles mosquito
    d. A vector-borne disease transmitted by the Aedes mosquito

18. Differentiate between inhalation and ingestion.
    a. Inhalation is the transmission of infectious disease through aerosolized germs, while ingestion is the transmission of infectious disease through body contact
    b. Inhalation is the transmission of infectious disease through aerosolized germs, while ingestion is the transmission of infectious disease through contaminated food or water
    c. Ingestion is the transmission of infectious disease through aerosolized germs, while inhalation is the transmission of the infectious disease through body contact
    d. Inhalation is the transmission of infectious disease through aerosolized germs, while ingestion is the transmission of the infectious disease through the nose

19. Where are aerosolized germs common?
    a. Medical equipment and construction sites
    b. Construction sites and chemical plants
    c. Chemical plants and quarries
    d. Gas stations and construction sites

20. Some direct infection transmission channels are:
    a. Sharing contaminated injection and syringes
    b. Human bites
    c. Hugging and kissing
    d. All of the above

21. What is an STD?
    a. A sexually transmission deformity
    b. A sexually transmitted deformity
    c. A sexually transmitted disease
    d. A sexually transmission disease

22. Some fungal diseases are:
    a. Sporothrix schenckii and fever
    b. Mycoses and runny nose
    c. Both A and B
    d. None of the above

23. Fungi are classified into:
    a. Yeasts, molds and dimorphic yeasts
    b. Molds, dibartic yeasts and dimorphic yeasts
    c. Simple and complex fungi
    d. Relative and abstract fungi

24. Which of the following diseases are transmitted by bacteria?
    a. Diphtheria, plague and typhoid
    b. Malaria, runny nose and fever
    c. Pneumonia, stool and infection
    d. Ringworm, tapeworm and cough

25. Parasites can gain entrance to the host's body through:
    a. Water and food
    b. Hair and skin
    c. Both A and B
    d. None of the above

26. Which of the following are examples of viral infections?
    a. Hepatitis, polio and dengue fever
    b. Malaria, typhoid and runny nose
    c. Stooling, malaria and typhoid
    d. Dengue fever, hepatitis and malaria

27. What is the proper order in the following chain?
    a. Fetus – embryo – zygote – baby
    b. Embryo – fetus – zygote – baby
    c. Zygote – embryo – fetus – baby
    d. Zygote – fetus – embryo – baby

28. What is erectile dysfunction?
    a. A medical condition that affects the female reproductive system
    b. A man's inability to get or sustain an erection for sexual intercourse
    c. A woman's inability to reach orgasm during sexual intercourse
    d. A medical condition that results in an inability for a woman to conceive

29. Which of the following is the most common medical condition associated with the male reproductive system?
    a. Erectile dysfunction
    b. Low sperm count
    c. Prostate cancer
    d. Cancer of the penis

30. Which of the following female reproductive system medical conditions is mild and can be treated with over-the-counter drugs?
    a. Pelvic inflammatory disease
    b. Endometriosis
    c. Yeast infection
    d. Menstrual cramping

31. Which of the following urinary system ailments is characterized by incomplete bladder emptying in men?
    a. Urinary tract infection
    b. Interstitial cystitis
    c. Incontinence
    d. Endometriosis

32. What is a urinary tract infection?
    a. A female-only urinary system problem that causes painful urination
    b. A male-only urinary system problem that causes painful urination
    c. A urinary system problem triggered by a bacterial attack on the urinary tract
    d. A urinary system problem triggered by a yeast attack on the urinary tract

33. What causes ejaculation?
    a. Ejaculation occurs when the bladder is filled with too much urine, leading to urine leakage
    b. Ejaculation refers to the release of waste products from the body, especially urine, from the bladder
    c. Ejaculation refers to the release of semen from the penis during sexual intercourse
    d. Ejaculation refers to the release of vaginal fluid due to the stimulation of the clitoris

34. What is the epididymis?
    a. A part of the central nervous system that controls most activities of the nervous system
    b. A part of the respiratory system that coordinates blood flow to the heart
    c. A part of the reproductive system where sperm undergoes development
    d. A special organ whose functions depend on the prevailing conditions

35. The male reproductive system performs all of the following functions except:
    a. Semen production
    b. Sex hormone production
    c. Semen released into the vagina during sexual intercourse
    d. Semen production and fertilization

36. Differentiate between the penis and the testicles.
    a. The testicles produce sperm cells, while the penis releases sperm cells into the vagina to fertilize the eggs
    b. The penis produces sperm cells, while the testicles release sperm cells into the vagina for fertilization
    c. The testicles produce sperm cells, while the penis releases fertilized sperm cells into the vagina
    d. The penis produces sperm cells, while the testicles release fertilized sperm cells into the vagina

37. What is the clitoris?
    a. The sensitive part of the male reproductive organ that responds to stimulation
    b. The sensitive part of the female reproductive organ that responds to stimulation
    c. The female reproductive organ where fertilization takes place
    d. The male reproductive organ where egg development takes place

38. The tube that serves as the channel between the bladder and the outside world is the:
    a. Bladder exit
    b. Bladder entry and exit point
    c. Urethra
    d. Nerves

39. What is the major difference between a ureter and a urethra?
    a. The urethra transports urine to the bladder from the kidneys, while the ureter passes urine from the bladder as waste during urination
    b. The ureter transports urine to the bladder from the kidneys, while the urethra passes urine from the bladder as waste during urination
    c. The urethra transports urine to the kidneys from the bladder, while the ureter passes urine from the bladder as waste during urination
    d. The ureter transports urine to the kidneys from the bladder, while the urethra passes urine from the bladder as waste during urination

40. In addition to balancing bodily fluids, what other function do the kidneys perform?
    a. They remove waste products and toxins from the body
    b. They aid digestion and metabolism
    c. They support the body's immune system
    d. They support blood flow to every part of the body

41. What are two major functions of the urinary system?
    a. Liquid waste elimination and regulating chemicals
    b. Liquid waste elimination and aiding digestion
    c. Aiding food digestion and promoting smooth waste product elimination
    d. Supporting the reproductive system

42. Which of the following is a medical condition that results in the kidneys' inability to concentrate?
    a. Nephrogenic diabetes contrite
    b. Nephrogenic diabetes insipidus
    c. Kidney infection
    d. Urinary kidney dysfunction syndrome

43. An infection of the kidneys is known as:
    a. Nephrotic syndrome
    b. Pyelonephritis
    c. Acute kidney failure
    d. Papillary necrosis

44. Inflammation of the airways is a symptom of which of the following?
    a. Bronchiectasis
    b. Asthma
    c. Cystic fibrosis
    d. Pleurisy

45. Arrhythmia is a medical condition that is characterized by which of the following?
    a. Abnormal heart rhythm
    b. Bloody and painful urination
    c. Diarrhea
    d. Aching joints

46. Lungs perform all of the following functions except:
    a. Respiration
    b. Absorption of water and alcohol
    c. Excretion of substances such as water and alcohol
    d. None of the above

47. The heart's chamber walls are different sizes, thanks to which of the following?
    a. Myocardium content of the walls
    b. Amount of fluid in the walls
    c. Amount of substances supported by the walls
    d. Varieties of functions performed by the walls

48. What serves as a metabolic agent for drugs?
    a. Heart
    b. Metabolic system
    c. Kidneys
    d. Liver

49. Which of the following is the brain's processing system?
    a. Frontal lobes
    b. Middle lobes
    c. Temporal lobes
    d. Occipital lobes

50. Sleeping and breathing are some activities performed by which part of the brain?
    a. The cerebellum
    b. The basal ganglia
    c. The brainstem
    d. The cortex

51. How many nerves does the human brain use for communication?
    a. Hundreds of nerves
    b. Thousands of nerves
    c. Billions of nerves
    d. A billion nerves

52. What is a function performed by the kidneys?
    a. Ensuring water balance
    b. Removing waste products and toxins from the body
    c. Controlling electrolyte balance
    d. All of the above

53. What is the size of the kidneys?
    a. About six inches long and approximately the size of a baby's head
    b. About five inches long and approximately the size of a large fist
    c. About ten inches long and approximately the size of a baby's head
    d. About ten inches long and approximately the size of a small fist

54. What are the five vital organs of the body?
    a. The kidneys, brain, liver, heart and lungs
    b. The brain, kidneys, liver, heart and eyes
    c. The ears, brain, kidneys, heart and nose
    d. The kidneys, liver, brain, lungs and eyes

55. What is the importance of considering emergency calls when scheduling appointments?
    a. It enables a physician to attend to urgent medical cases promptly
    b. It is proof of a physician's efficiency
    c. It shows that patients can obtain medical attention and care at their convenience
    d. It is proof of a physician's respect for medical ethics

56. How do you schedule an appointment for a habitually late patient?
    a. Give the person the first appointment of the day
    b. Schedule the appointment for the afternoon
    c. Give the person the last appointment of the day
    d. Give the person multiple appointments in a day

57. What is an appointment reminder?
    a. A member of staff who reminds a physician about appointments
    b. A software program that reminds physicians about appointments
    c. A medical assistant responsible for scheduling and reminding physicians of appointments
    d. A calendar with appointments marked on it

58. When prioritizing appointments, which of the following factors must you consider?
    a. Patients' diverse needs
    b. Patients' work schedule
    c. Patients' health condition and availability
    d. The urgency of patients' individual medical conditions

59. In advanced scheduling, how much advance notice are patients required to give if they must cancel an appointment?
    a. 12 hours
    b. 24 hours
    c. 36 hours
    d. 48 hours

60. What is the difference between open office hours and flexible office hours?
    a. Open office hours are during the week, while flexible office hours are on weekends or evenings
    b. Flexible office hours are during the week, while open office hours are on weekends or evenings
    c. Open office hours last for 12 hours, while flexible office hours are undefined
    d. Flexible office hours are during the week, while open office hours are undefined

61. What appointment type enables a physician to attend to patients on a first-come, first-served basis?
    a. Wave scheduling
    b. Open office hours
    c. Advanced scheduling
    d. Flexible office hours

62. What factor must you consider when assigning a time length for an appointment?
    a. The amount of time the appointment will take the physician
    b. The distance between the patient's home and the medical facility
    c. How much free time a physician has on his/her schedule
    d. A wide range of factors that include existing weather conditions

63. Which of the following factors does not determine a patient's needs?
    a. The patient's work schedule
    b. How long it will take the patient to get to the medical facility
    c. The patient's physical condition
    d. The patient's economic status

64. Which of the following is not included when considering a physician's preferences for appointments?
    a. Having a scheduled break at regular intervals
    b. Phone calls
    c. Chart examinations
    d. Time for reading medical texts

65. Which of the following is not a type of appointment scheduling?
    a. Advanced scheduling
    b. Open office hours
    c. Wave scheduling
    d. Interference scheduling

66. What is the largest part of the human brain?
    a. Cerebrum
    b. Cerebellum
    c. Ventricles
    d. Cavities

67. What is the outermost layer of the brain?
    a. The brainstem
    b. The basal ganglia
    c. The cerebellum
    d. None of the above

68. What controls hearing and memory?
    a. The frontal and occipital lobes
    b. The temporal and frontal lobes
    c. Both A and B
    d. None of the above

69. Which are not components of the liver?
    a. Gallbladder and intestines
    b. Pancreas and intestines
    c. Gallbladder and pancreas
    d. Intestines and ventricles

70. Which part of the body secretes bile?
    a. The left lung
    b. The liver
    c. The heart
    d. The kidneys

71. What makes up the heart's outer layer?
    a. Endocardium
    b. Epicardium
    c. Myocardium
    d. None of the above

72. Differentiate between systemic veins and pulmonary veins.
    a. Pulmonary veins pass deoxygenated blood to the right atrium, while systemic veins pass oxygenated blood to the left atrium
    b. Systemic veins pass deoxygenated blood to the right atrium, while pulmonary veins pass oxygenated blood to the left atrium
    c. Pulmonary veins pass deoxygenated blood to the left atrium, while systemic veins pass oxygenated blood to the right atrium
    d. Systemic veins pass deoxygenated blood to the left atrium, while pulmonary veins pass oxygenated blood to the right atrium

73. The lungs are covered with a thin tissue layer known as:
    a. Pleura
    b. Bronchiole
    c. Alveoli
    d. Lobules

74. An active person uses how much of his/her lungs' gaseous exchange surface?
    a. One-tenth
    b. One-fifth
    c. One-twentieth
    d. One-third

75. Which of the following are non-infectious causes of hepatitis?
    a. Heavy drinking and allergic reactions
    b. Drugs and obesity
    c. Allergic reactions and drugs
    d. All of the above

76. What is the major difference between cirrhosis and hemochromatosis?
    a. Cirrhosis is temporary liver damage, while hemochromatosis is permanent liver damage
    b. Hemochromatosis is temporary liver damage, while cirrhosis is permanent liver damage
    c. Cirrhosis is permanent liver damage, while hemochromatosis occurs when iron is deposited in the liver
    d. Hemochromatosis is permanent liver damage, while cirrhosis occurs when iron is deposited in the liver

77. Differentiate between arrhythmia and dysrhythmia.
    a. Arrhythmia causes an abnormal heart rhythm, while dysrhythmia refers to abnormal inflammation of the kidneys
    b. Dysrhythmia causes abnormal inflammation of the kidneys, while arrhythmia refers to an abnormal rhythm of the kidneys' urine excretion
    c. Arrhythmia causes abnormal heart pounding, while dysrhythmia refers to an abnormal inflammation of the left lung
    d. Arrhythmia and dysrhythmia are synonyms

78. An inflammation of the pericardium can result in a medical condition known as which of the following?
    a. Pericarditis inflammation syndrome
    b. Pericarditis inflammation and infection syndrome
    c. Pericarditis
    d. Pericarditis infection and inflammation syndrome

79. Clogging of the kidneys due to damaged kidney tissues is the primary cause of which of the following?
    a. Nephrogenic diabetes insipidus
    b. Papillary necrosis
    c. Nephrotic syndrome
    d. Pyelonephritis

80. How is urrea formed?
    a. The breakdown of protein-rich foods
    b. The breakdown of carbohydrate-rich foods
    c. Essential minerals and vitamins
    d. All of the above

81. What can cause a kidney infection?
    a. Excessive consumption of salty foods
    b. Excessive consumption of sugar-rich foods and drinks
    c. Holding urine for too long
    d. Smoking

82. What role do the sphincter muscles play in the urinary system?
    a. They prevent accidental blood flow through the urinary tract
    b. They prevent accidental urine leakage
    c. They ensure easy urination
    d. They remove impurities from the urinary tract

83. Which are produced regularly to sustain the reproductive cycle?
    a. Male sex hormones
    b. Female sex hormones
    c. Hormones and chromosomes
    d. Hormones and zygotes

84. Which of the following reproductive roles is not the vagina's responsibility?
    a. Sperm cell production
    b. Sexual intercourse
    c. Blood passage during menstruation
    d. None of the above

85. Which of the following are not attributes of the hymen?
    a. It covers the vagina's opening
    b. Hymens are different from one woman to another
    c. Hymens are always broken during the first sexual intercourse
    d. Hymens are thin tissues

86. What are the dimensions of an average womb?
    a. Three inches wide and two inches long
    b. Four inches wide and eight inches long
    c. Two inches wide and three inches long
    d. Three inches wide and four inches long

87. Which part of the female reproductive organs carries urine from the bladder through the vagina?
    a. Labia majora
    b. Labie minora
    c. Labie majora
    d. Labia minora

88. Where do the two labia minora meet?
   a. Clitoris
   b. Vagina
   c. Uterus wall
   d. Prepuce

89. What are the major components of the accessory glands?
   a. Prostate gland and seminal vesicles
   b. Prostate gland and seminal container
   c. Seminal vesicles and duct system
   d. The testicles and seminal vesicles

90. How many sperm does an adult male produce at puberty?
   a. Millions of sperm cells monthly
   b. Millions of sperm cells daily
   c. Millions of sperm cells weekly
   d. Millions of sperm cells annually

91. After complete development, sperm is transported from the epididymis to:
   a. The vas deferens
   b. The seminal vesicles
   c. The prostate gland
   d. None of the above

92. How many sperm are released during each ejaculation?
   a. Tens of thousands
   b. About 100 million
   c. About 500 million
   d. About 50 thousand

93. Which of the following are common symptoms of interstitial cystitis?
   a. Bladder scarring and hampered elasticity
   b. Hampered elasticity and bladder shrinking
   c. A defect in the patient's stomach lining
   d. All of the above

94. Pelvic inflammatory disease is caused by which of the following sexually transmitted diseases?
    a. HIV and syphilis
    b. Gonorrhea and chlamydia
    c. Gonorrhea and syphilis
    d. Chlamydia and HIV

95. What can treat prostate cancer?
    a. Hormonal treatment
    b. Radiation therapy
    c. Watchful waiting
    d. All of the above

96. What is a fertilized egg?
    a. A zygote
    b. An embryo
    c. A fetus
    d. None of the above

97. Plague, cholera and dysentery are examples of diseases transmitted by which of the following?
    a. Fungi
    b. Bacteria
    c. Virus
    d. Parasites

98. Blastomyces dermatitidis and Histoplasma capsulatum are examples of diseases that can be transmitted by which of the following?
    a. Bacteria
    b. Vectors
    c. Parasites
    d. Fungi

99. Which of the following are not a part of the chain of infection?
    a. Pathogens and portal of exit
    b. Portal of entry and new host
    c. Portal of entry and portal of dissemination
    d. Reservoir and means of transmission

100. How should waste be disposed of?

a. Leak-proof bag with appropriate biohazard symbol
b. Durable bag with appropriate color markings
c. Transparent and lightweight bag
d. Leak-proof and lightweight bag

Practice Test 4 – Answers

1) **d:** Four

There are four vital signs that are the most basic functions of the body. These are blood pressure, temperature, respiratory rate and pulse rate.

2) **b:** 36.5°C and 37.2°C

A healthy person's body temperature ranges between 36.5°C and 37.2°C or between 97.8°F and 99°F. A temperature above that range is a symptom of fever.

3) **a:** It is cost-effective and improves health

Treatment compliance is cost-effective and enhances the chances of improved health. Patients do not have to spend more money or focus on treating a relapse.

4) **a:** Weight and height

When conducting a physical examination on a patient, a medical professional should measure height and weight. He/she should also look for deformities or irregularities in the patient's body. Such findings should be recorded and passed along to the physician in charge of the patient.

5) **d:** None of the above

Subjective data are a set of information provided by a patient to help the physician determine a person's ailments and the correct treatment. Some examples of subjective data are dizziness, coughing, itching, shortness of breath, vomiting and exhaustion.

6) **d:** Vomiting and dizziness

Objective data are visible to the physician. They include height and weight, heart rate, blood pressure, general appearance and body temperature. They are essential metrics for all patients.

7) **b:** The patient's major complaint

While health workers may collect a variety of information that gives insight into a patient's medical condition, they must first listen to the patient's complaint. The complaint gives an idea of how the patient feels. This is useful information for the physician.

8) **b:** Past medical history

One of the most important questions that can help a physician to understand a patient's medical history is, "What ailment have you been treated for recently?" This is important because the patient's medical history is a component of the medical record.

9) **d:** All of the above

Fomites are inanimate objects through which infectious diseases can be transmitted to healthy people. Some examples of fomites are sinks, rails, toilets, doorknobs, door handles and bus seats.

10) **a:** When a medical worker is at high risk of being contaminated by bodily fluids

Medical workers can protect themselves against infections in a number of ways, including wearing appropriate protective equipment, such as goggles and surgical masks.

11) **b:** An alcohol-based solution

Soiled hands are best washed with an alcohol-based solution. However, for general hand cleaning, washing with soap and water is sufficient. Alcohol sanitizers are equally good for hand cleaning.

12) **b:** When you touch a contaminated object, even if you wear gloves

Handwashing ranks among the most effective way to guard against infection. Wash your hands whenever you touch a contaminated object with bare hands, when you feel it is necessary to do so and when you feel symptoms of an infection.

13) **a:** Genetic makeup

The genetic makeup of a host determines its resistance to infection. For instance, someone with sickle-cell traits will be more susceptible to infections than others.

14) **b:** A new host

A new host is the final link in the chain of infection. There are six links in the chain of infection: pathogen, reservoir, portal of exit, means of transmission, portal of entry and new host, in that order.

15) **b:** The channel through which a transmission agent enters the host's body

The portal of entry refers to the means through which a pathogen enters its host. This may be through inhalation, penetration or ingestion. It may also be through the mucous membranes, as seen in syphilis; through the skin, as seen in hookworm; or through the blood.

16) **a:** Saliva and urine

When contaminated food is chewed, eaten, swallowed or licked, the virus will be transmitted through a person's saliva. Exudates, urine and feces are some types of contaminants.

17) **d:** A vector-borne disease transmitted by the Aedes mosquito

Yellow fever is a vector-borne disease transmitted by the Aedes mosquito. Other vector-borne diseases are malaria, dengue fever, Lyme disease, Chagas and lymphatic filariasis.

18) **b:** Inhalation is the transmission of infectious disease through aerosolized germs, while ingestion is the transmission of infectious disease through contaminated food or water

Inhalation and ingestion are two of the major modes of infection transmission. However, while inhalation refers to the transmission of infectious disease through aerosolized germs, ingestion refers to the consumption of contaminated food or water.

19) **a:** Medical equipment and construction sites

Sometimes, medical equipment contains aerosolized germs. Such germs are also a common feature in construction zones, where dust serves as their host. Aspergillus or nontuberculous mycobacteria are transmitted through this medium.

20) **d:** All of the above

Some direct infection transmission channels are kissing, hugging and human bites. Sharing syringes and contaminated needles is another means of direct infection transmission. Generally, any physical contact between a carrier and a healthy person can lead to infection transmission.

21) **c:** A sexually transmitted disease

STD means sexually transmitted disease. These are medical conditions that are transmitted via sexual intercourse. Examples of STDs are HIV/AIDS, syphilis and gonorrhea.

22) **d:** None of the above

Fungi are the cause of diseases such as athlete's foot and ringworm. Mycoses, histoplasmosis, aspergillosis and Coccidioidomycosis are some fungal diseases. Sporothrix schenckii, runny nose and fever are not fungal diseases.

23) **a:** Yeasts, molds and dimorphic yeasts

There are different types of fungi. Some are molds, yeasts and dimorphic yeasts. Fungi are some of the most destructive infectious agents. They are ubiquitous and transport several ailments from one person to another.

24) **a:** Diphtheria, plague and typhoid

Bacteria have contributed immensely to the transfer of diseases that have claimed millions of lives. History shows that these pathogens are the hosts for deadly diseases, such as bacterial pneumonia, diphtheria, tuberculosis and typhoid. They are also the carriers for cholera, plague and dysentery.

25) **c:** Both A and B

Parasites are living organisms whose existence depends on another living organism. They are mostly disease carriers and may undermine their hosts' health. Some parasites gain entrance to the host's body through contaminated water or food, while some live on the host's hair or skin.

26) **a:** Hepatitis, polio and dengue

Herpes, rabies, Ebola and COVID-19 are some types of viral infections. Others are measles, hepatitis, dengue fever, HIV, hepatitis and polio.

27) **c:** Zygote – embryo – fetus – baby

A fertilized egg is referred to as a zygote. The zygote undergoes repeated divisions as it grows in the uterus. It matures first into an embryo, and subsequently into a fetus until it grows into a baby ready for delivery.

28) **b:** A man's inability to get or sustain an erection for sexual intercourse

Erectile dysfunction is a medical condition in which a man cannot get an erection or is unable to sustain an erection for sexual intercourse. According to some medical experts, almost one out of every ten males experiences the chronic and untreatable form of this ailment.

29) **c:** Prostate cancer

Prostate cancer is a medical condition of the male reproductive system. It affects the small gland that produces the seminal fluid used for nourishing and transporting sperm. It is the most common disease that affects the male reproductive organs and can result in an array of medical conditions such as frequent urination.

30) **c:** Yeast infection

This is a disease of the reproductive system common in females. As the name implies, it can be traced to a yeast fungus found in the vagina. This condition can usually be treated easily with over-the-counter drugs.

31) **c:** Incontinence

This medical condition is common to the urinary system. Patients with this ailment usually have the urge to urinate frequently. Male patients usually struggle with incomplete bladder emptying due to the enlargement of the prostate.

32) **c:** A urinary system problem triggered by a bacterial attack on the urinary tract

This occurs in the urinary system when the urinary tract is affected by bacteria. The bacteria can affect several organs, such as the bladder, urethra and kidneys. According to the American Urological Association, over eight million Americans suffer from this ailment.

33) **c:** Ejaculation refers to the release of semen from the penis during sexual intercourse

Sexual intercourse increases the stimulation of the erect penis. This forces the contraction of the muscles surrounding the reproductive organs. As the contraction continues, semen is forced out through the urethra and the duct system via a process known as ejaculation.

34) **c:** A part of the reproductive system where sperm undergoes development

Sperm cells undergo division and transformation until each assumes a tadpole-like structure with a short tail and head. The sperm will subsequently relocate to the epididymis, where they will undergo complete development. After they have developed completely, sperm are transported to the vas deferens, or sperm duct.

35) **d:** Semen production and fertilization

The male reproductive system produces semen. It releases semen into a female's reproductive system during sexual intercourse through ejaculation. It also produces sex hormones at puberty.

36) **a:** The testicles produce sperm cells, while the penis releases sperm into the vagina to fertilize the eggs

The penis and testicles are major components of the male reproductive system. The testicles produce sperm cells, while the penis releases the sperm into the vagina to fertilize the eggs.

37) **b:** The sensitive part of the female reproductive organ that responds to stimulation

The clitoris is the meeting point for the two labia minora. It is a small but very sensitive part of the female reproductive organs that protrudes in a manner that draws comparisons between it and a male penis, especially when it is fully stimulated.

38) **c:** Urethra

The urethra is a tube that serves as the channel between the urine in the bladder and the outside world. The bladder receives signals from the brain to tighten and thereby squeeze and push the urine through the urethra.

39) **b:** The ureter transports urine to the bladder from the kidneys, while the urethra passes urine from the bladder as waste during urination

The urinary system is made up of the ureter, urethra and other components. Urine transportation from the kidneys to the bladder is handled by the ureter, while the urethra supports the transportation of urine from the bladder as waste during urination.

40) **a:** They remove waste products and toxins from the body

Kidneys remove waste products and toxins from the body. In addition, they ensure water balance, control blood pressure and regulate electrolyte levels.

41) **a:** Liquid waste elimination and regulating chemicals

The urinary system is responsible for eliminating liquids from the body in the form of urine. It also regulates some body chemicals.

42) **b:** Nephrogenic diabetes insipidus

This medical condition, triggered by a drug reaction, occurs when the kidneys can no longer concentrate the urine. Although this health problem may be mild, it can cause frequent urination and constant thirst.

43) **b:** Pyelonephritis

This is also known as a kidney infection. This health problem is triggered by bacteria in the kidneys. This condition may result in fever or back pain.

44) **b:** Asthma

Asthma is a chronic disease characterized by the inflammation and swelling of the bronchial tubes' lining. It usually causes difficulty breathing. Asthma is a chronic disease that requires special medical attention to manage.

45) **a:** Abnormal heart rhythm

Arrhythmia is also known as dysrhythmia. This medical condition is an abnormal heart rhythm that occurs when the conduction of electrical impulses via the heart is disrupted. Some cases of this medical condition may be mild, while some are life-threatening.

46) **d:** None of the above

The lungs are primarily designed for respiratory activities. In addition to that, they absorb alcohol and water.

47) **a:** Myocardium content of the walls

The heart's chamber walls are different sizes. The differences are caused by the different amounts of myocardium in the heart, a reflection of the amount of force that must be generated by each chamber.

48) **d:** Liver

The liver is made up of components, such as the gallbladder, pancreas and intestines. They enable it to perform several functions, such as serving as a metabolic agent for drugs. It also serves as a detoxification agent for chemicals so that the body can assimilate ingested chemicals and drugs.

49) **d:** Occipital lobes

The occipital lobes are the center of the brain's processing ability.

50) **c:** The brainstem

The brainstem is an important part of the brain. It controls various body systems, specifically breathing and sleeping.

51) **c:** Billions of nerves

The brain is the control center of the entire body, thanks to its more than 100 billion nerves that use trillions of synapses for communication.

52) **d:** All of the above

The kidneys ensure water balance in the body, remove waste products and toxins, and regulate electrolyte balance. They release hormones that are needed for blood pressure control. They control phosphorus and calcium, supporting bone health.

53) **b:** About five inches long and approximately the size of a large fist

On either side of the spine is a kidney, a bean-shaped internal body organ. Each kidney is located behind the belly and below the ribs. Each kidney is about five inches long and is approximately the size of a large fist.

54) **a:** The kidneys, brain, liver, heart and lungs

The five vital organs of the body are the liver, brain, kidneys, heart and lungs. Individually, they play important roles in the body. Collectively, they are crucial to the body's overall health.

55) **a:** It enables a physician to attend to urgent medical cases promptly

When scheduling appointments, factors that must be considered include emergency calls. Creating room for emergency calls enables a physician to attend to urgent medical cases promptly without disrupting treatment for other patients already on the schedule for the day.

56) **c:** Give the person the last appointment of the day

If a patient is constantly late, give him/her the last appointment of the day. That way, if he/she arrives late, it will not create a problem with the doctor's other scheduled appointments.

57) **b:** A software program that reminds physicians about appointments

Appointment reminders ensure that physicians are kept apprised of their upcoming appointments in a timely fashion.

58) **a:** Patients' diverse needs

Patients' needs are diverse. Thus, the degree of time you need to attend to their individual needs differs as well. When scheduling appointments, it is important that you take these kinds of factors into consideration.

59) **b:** 24 hours

In some cases of advanced scheduling, some physicians require that they receive 24 hours' notice if the patient wants to cancel the appointment. This ensures that a vacant appointment time is not wasted.

60) **a:** Open office hours are during the week, while flexible office hours are on weekends or evenings

Appointments that are scheduled during the week are attended to during open office hours, while those booked for evenings or weekends are flexible office-hour appointments.

61) **a:** Wave scheduling

Wave scheduling offers some flexibility. It involves planning a specific number of appointments within a specific period of time. Thus, a doctor can attend to patients in order of their arrival.

62) **a:** The amount of time the appointment will take the physician

When assigning a time frame for an appointment, consider the amount of time it may take the physician. You will cause a doctor great scheduling difficulties if you book 20 minutes for a procedure that may take an hour.

63) **d:** The patient's economic status

A patient's needs are based on several factors. The patient's work schedule, the distance between the medical facility and the patient's place of residence, and the patient's physical condition are important factors. The patient's economic status is irrelevant.

64) **d:** Time for reading medical texts

A physician's preference takes several factors into consideration. This includes having breaks at intervals during working hours, time to make and receive phone calls and time to examine charts and other documents. Time for reading medical texts does not factor in.

65) **d:** Interference scheduling

There are different types of scheduling: wave scheduling, open office hours, advanced scheduling, flexible office hours and scheduled appointments. Interference scheduling does not exist.

66) **a:** Cerebrum

The cerebrum forms the largest part of the brain.

67) **d:** None of the above

The outermost layer of the brain is called the cerebral cortex. Therefore, none of the options in the question can be the outermost layer of the brain.

68) **d:** None of the above

Only temporal lobes control memory and hearing. Frontal lobes handle an individual's problem-solving abilities, and the occipital lobes are the brain's visual processing system.

69) **d:** Intestines and ventricles

The gallbladder, intestines and pancreas work together with the liver to perform multiple functions, such as food digestion, absorption and processing. Ventricles are not organs of the liver.

70) **b:** The liver

In addition to filtering blood, the liver also secretes bile that eventually ends up in the intestines. This greenish-brown and bitter fluid is stored in the gall bladder, and it aids digestion.

71) **b:** Epicardium

The outer layer of the heart is epicardium. The myocardium is the middle layer, while the endocardium makes up the inner layer. These three layers form the heart's wall.

72) **b:** Systemic veins pass deoxygenated blood to the right atrium, while pulmonary veins pass oxygenated blood to the left atrium

Both systemic veins and pulmonary veins pass blood to the atrium. The right atrium receives deoxygenated blood from the systemic veins, while the left atrium is supplied with oxygenated blood by the pulmonary veins.

73) **a:** Pleura

The pleura is a thin tissue layer that covers the lungs. This type of thin tissue also lines the external part of the chest cavity.

74) **c:** One-twentieth

If you are active, you only use about one-twentieth of the lung's gaseous-exchange surface. As your engagement in vigorous physical activity increases, the portion of the surface you use increases correspondingly.

75) **d:** All of the above

Hepatitis is an inflammation of the liver. The medical condition can be caused by infection and non-infectious factors. The non-infectious causes are drugs, heavy drinking, allergic reactions and obesity.

76) **c:** Cirrhosis is permanent liver damage, while hemochromatosis occurs when iron is deposited in the liver

The liver is prone to many medical conditions. Two of them are hemochromatosis and cirrhosis. While the former is caused by iron deposited in the liver, the latter refers to permanent damage of the vital organ.

77) **d:** Arrhythmia and dysrhythmia are synonyms

Arrhythmia is an abnormal heart rhythm that occurs when the conduction of electrical impulses via the heart is altered. Some cases of this medical condition may be mild, while some are life-threatening. This medical condition is also known as dysrhythmia.

78) **d:** Pericarditis

Inflammation of the pericardium can result in a medical condition known as pericarditis. Some common causes of the heart problem include kidney failure, viral infection and autoimmune conditions.

79) **b:** Papillary necrosis

When the kidneys are severely damaged, the kidney tissues may break internally, thereby clogging the kidneys. If this condition is left untreated, it will aggravate the condition, worsening the damage already done. That may result in papillary necrosis or total kidney failure.

80) **a:** The breakdown of protein-rich foods

When someone consumes protein-rich foods, such as poultry and meat, they are broken down in the individual's body to form urea. The waste is subsequently transported to the kidneys through the blood. The urea and other waste are removed from the body as urine.

81) **c:** Holding urine for too long

The body informs you of the need to urinate through the bladder nerves. If you ignore this sign and hold your urine for too long, you run the risk of getting a kidney infection.

82) **b:** They prevent accidental urine leakage

The sphincter muscles receive signals from the brain to relax and allow the urine easy passage through the urethra.

83) **b:** Female sex hormones

The reproductive cycle is a continuous process for women of child-bearing age. To keep the cycle going, the female reproductive system produces female sex hormones regularly.

84) **a:** Sperm cell production

The vagina plays several roles in the female reproductive system. Sperm cell production is not one of them. The male reproductive system is responsible for producing sperm cells needed to fertilize the eggs produced by the female reproductive system.

85) **c:** Hymens are always broken during the first sexual intercourse

The vagina's opening is covered by a thin tissue, the hymen. This differs from one woman to another. Hymens are most often broken during the first sexual experience, while some women have theirs broken even before their first sexual encounter.

86) **c:** Two inches wide and three inches long

The womb has muscular walls and a thick lining. The muscles are stronger than most muscles in a female and can contract and expand, allowing a fetus enough space to grow without harm. In a woman who is not pregnant, the uterus is about two inches wide and three inches long.

87) **d:** Labia minora

The labia minora are about two inches wide. They are inside the labia majora, surrounding the urethra.

88) **a:** Clitoris

The two labia minora meet at the clitoris. This is a very sensitive part of the female reproductive system, which responds to stimulation in a manner reminiscent of the penis.

89) **a:** Prostate gland and seminal vesicles

The accessory glands include the prostate gland and the seminal vesicles. These organs provide the fluids needed by the duct system for lubrication. The sperm is also nourished with the fluids.

90) **b:** Millions of sperm daily

An adult male at puberty produces millions of sperm cells daily. These are tiny cells about 0.05 millimeters long. The sperm develops in the seminiferous tubules located in the testicles.

91) **a:** The vas deferens

Sperm cells are produced by a male at puberty. The cells are transformed and divided until each assumes a tadpole-like structure. The sperm will subsequently relocate to the epididymis, where they will undergo complete development. After they have developed completely, they are transported to the vas deferens, or sperm duct.

92) **c:** About 500 million

Ejaculation occurs when the semen exits through the urethra. With each ejaculation, some 500 million sperm are released.

93) **d:** All of the above

Some common symptoms of interstitial cystitis are bladder scarring, hampered elasticity, bladder shrinking and a defect in the patient's bladder lining. This medical condition is common in women and can cause untold bladder pressure and pain. Hence, it is also known as painful bladder syndrome.

94) **b:** Gonorrhea and chlamydia

Pelvic inflammatory disease refers to an infection that affects any of the reproductive organs in females. This may include the ovaries and the uterus. The medical condition can be traced to sexually transmitted diseases, such as chlamydia and gonorrhea. Aside from pelvic inflammatory disease, these STIs can also trigger infertility.

95) **d:** All of the above

Prostate cancer is a medical condition of the male reproductive system. It affects the small gland that produces the seminal fluid used for nourishing and transporting sperm. Hormonal treatment, radiation therapy and watchful waiting are some effective treatment options for the ailment.

96) **a:** A zygote
Millions of sperm swim from the vagina through the uterus and the cervix into the fallopian tubes to meet the newly released egg and fertilize it. The fertilized egg is called a zygote, consisting of 46 chromosomes; 23 from each of the egg and the sperm.

97) **b:** Bacteria

Plague, cholera and dysentery are examples of some diseases transferred by bacteria. These pathogens are also the hosts for bacterial pneumonia, diphtheria, tuberculosis and typhoid.

98) **d:** Fungi

Blastomyces dermatitidis and Histoplasma capsulatum are some diseases transmitted by fungi. Fungi also cause athlete's foot and ringworm. Mycoses, histoplasmosis, aspergillosis and Coccidioidomycosis arc some fungal diseases.

99) **c:** Portal of entry and portal of dissemination

Portal of entry and portal of dissemination are not part of the chain of infection. The chain includes pathogens, reservoir, portal of exit, portal of entry, a new host and means of transmission.

100) **a:** Leak-proof bag with appropriate biohazard symbol

Waste should be disposed of in a leak-proof bag with an appropriate biohazard symbol.

Practice Test 5

1. Food is classified into how many classes?
    a. Six
    b. Five
    c. Three
    d. Ten

2. Dietary carbohydrates are divided into what?
    a. Sugars, starches and fiber
    b. Starches, fiber and essential elements
    c. Fiber, sugars and essential elements
    d. Essential elements, sugar and fiber

3. Which of the following groups of foods is rich in protein?
    a. Meat, beans and nuts
    b. Meat, beans and fish
    c. Fish, eggs and meat
    d. Soy, meat and egg

4. What are saturated fats?
    a. Fats with high amounts of hydrogen atoms
    b. Fats with high amounts of carbon atoms
    c. Fats with high amounts of oxygen atoms
    d. Fats with high amounts of hydrogen and carbon atoms

5. Which of the following are examples of polyunsaturated fats?
    a. Oysters, sunflower seeds and salmon
    b. Herring, peanuts and sunflower
    c. Avocados, mackerel and sunflower seeds
    d. Sardines, peanut oil and mackerel

6. What are some good sources of water-soluble vitamins?
    a. Vitamin C, vitamin B3 and vitamin B12
    b. Vitamin A, vitamin B9 and vitamin B1
    c. Vitamin B4, vitamin B3 and vitamin B9
    d. Vitamin A, vitamin B4 and vitamin C

7. Vitamin deficiencies can result in the following medical conditions:
    a. Fever, beriberi and rickets
    b. Beriberi, typhoid and rickets
    c. Ulcers, pellagra and beriberi
    d. Pellagra, rickets and typhoid

8. Weight management can be achieved by consuming all of the following foods except:
    a. Beans and legumes
    b. Leafy greens and whole grains
    c. Fruits and legumes
    d. White rice and white bread

9. What is a medical condition that can trigger a stroke?
    a. Low blood pressure
    b. High blood pressure
    c. Carbohydrate deficiency
    d. Protein deficiency

10. Why are cancer patients prone to malnutrition?
    a. They do not consume carbohydrates
    b. They do not eat protein-rich foods
    c. They lose their appetite
    d. Chemotherapy may cause malnutrition

11. What is lactose?
    a. A type of sugar found in sugary fruits
    b. A type of sugar found in carbohydrates
    c. A type of sugar found in sugar-rich canned foods
    d. A type of sugar found in animal milk

12. What is binge-eating disorder?
    a. A disorder characterized by an unusual appetite
    b. A disorder characterized by a reduced appetite
    c. A disorder that is characterized by an unusual appetite for starchy food
    d. A disorder characterized by an unusual appetite for vegetables and fruits

13. What is specimen collection?
    a. The process of collecting specimens for use in the laboratory during titration
    b. The process of collecting tissues or fluids for laboratory analysis
    c. The collection of bodily fluids during a pregnancy test
    d. The collection of blood during a genotype test

14. What is the importance of specimen collection?
    a. It guarantees cheaper treatment and diagnosis
    b. It guarantees accurate diagnosis and treatment
    c. It helps patients understand their medical condition
    d. It assists with medical record updating

15. What are some blood-taking techniques?
    a. Venipuncture and dermal analysis
    b. Dermal analysis and venecuture
    c. Dermal puncture and venipuncture
    d. None of the above

16. Random specimen refers to which of the following?
    a. A blood specimen that can be taken at any time of the day
    b. A blood specimen that can be taken at random intervals
    c. A urine specimen that can be taken only in the morning and at night
    d. A urine specimen that can be taken at any time of the day

17. What are some medical conditions that can require a sputum test?
    a. Fatigue and body aches
    b. Breathing difficulties and coughing
    c. Both A and B
    d. None of the above

18. How are analytical errors detected in the laboratory?
    a. Analytical error detection mechanism
    b. Laboratory quality control
    c. Laboratory error control process
    d. Analytical quality and error control

19. Which branch of science deals with the study of drugs and their effects on consumers?
    a. Pharmacy
    b. Pharmacology
    c. Pharmacist
    d. Pharmacologist

20. Drugs are classified into how many classes?
    a. Seven
    b. Five
    c. Three
    d. Ten

21. What are depressants?
    a. Drugs that are recommended for boosting libido
    b. Drugs to correct pregnancy issues in women
    c. Drugs that affect the central nervous system
    d. Drugs that regulate the frequency of urination

22. What are some permanent effects of depressants?
    a. Chronic breathing difficulties and high body temperature
    b. Sexual problems and chronic fatigue
    c. Both A and B
    d. None of the above

23. What are short-term effects of stimulants?
    a. Exhaustion and depression
    b. Increased appetite and fever
    c. Loss of appetite and depression
    d. Exhaustion and allergies

24. What are aerosol sprays used for?
    a. They are used as stimulants
    b. They are used as inhalants
    c. They are used as libido boosters
    d. They are used as hormone regulators

25. What are two short-term effects of inhalants?
    a. Lack of coordination and distorted speech
    b. Dizziness and mental fatigue
    c. Euphoria and addiction
    d. Liver damage and hearing loss

26. What are hallucinogens?
    a. A group of drugs that cause cancer in women
    b. A group of drugs that cause cancer in men
    c. A group of drugs that cause anomalies and changes in consciousness
    d. A group of drugs that cause permanent hearing loss

27. What are two common hallucinogens?
    a. Psilocybin and mescaline
    b. LSC and mescaline
    c. Tetrapine and mescaline
    d. Psilocybin and depressonite

28. Regular cannabis use can trigger all of the following medical conditions except:
    a. Selective impairment of cognitive function
    b. Reduction in birth weight
    c. Impairment of several body organs
    d. None of the above

29. Differentiate between opioids and cannabis.
    a. Opioids are used to cure respiratory problems, while cannabis regulates heartbeat
    b. Cannabis is used to cure respiratory problems, while opioids regulate heartbeat
    c. Cannabis is a mood-altering drug, while opioids relieve pain in the nervous system
    d. Opioids are mood-altering drugs, while cannabis relieves pain in the nervous system.

30. What is the major determinant factor for drug storage?
    a. The cost of the drug
    b. The major functions of the drug
    c. Storage instructions from the manufacturer
    d. Available storage facilities

31. What is the ideal temperature for storing medications marked "refrigerated"?
    a. Between 2 and 8°C
    b. Between 25 and 35°C
    c. Between 15 and 27°C
    d. Between 25 and 30°C

32. What are some general storage conditions for all types of medicine?
    a. They should be stored in a dry, cool place and away from children
    b. They should be stored in a humid place and away from children
    c. They should be stored at room temperature and away from children
    d. They should be stored in a warm, humid place and within reach

33. Dangerous or unexpected reactions to a drug are known as:
    a. Side effects
    b. Drug side impacts
    c. Adverse drug reactions
    d. Drug unwanted reactions

34. Congenital abnormalities, death and disabilities are consequences of which of the following?
    a. Drug overdose
    b. Drug addiction
    c. Severe adverse drug reaction
    d. Chronic addiction to drugs

35. What is the *Physicians' Desk Reference*?
    a. It is a reference document for easy access to appointments and patients' data
    b. It is an ergonomic desk
    c. It is a list of referrals for emergency medical attention
    d. It is a special annual reference guide for physicians

36. The *Physicians' Desk Reference* includes which of the following?
    a. Contact information for state DEA programs
    b. Controlled substance categories
    c. Drug dosage and indications
    d. All of the above

37. What does Section 2 of the *Physicians' Desk Reference* contain?
    a. Manufacturer's address and page numbers of where you can find additional information on specific subjects
    b. Generic name and pagination
    c. Product identification and product category index
    d. Information provided by manufacturers' names arranged alphabetically

38. What is first aid?
    a. The first financial assistance a medical facility receives from the government annually
    b. The initial medical assistance provided to a patient before the arrival of higher-level medical care
    c. The initial payment made by a patient before the commencement of treatment.
    d. The first treatment a patient receives in a series of treatments

39. What is the first approach to stop bleeding?
    a. Raise the affected part above the heart to slow the bleeding down
    b. Apply pressure to the affected area with a clean cloth
    c. Place ice on the affected area to stop the blood flow
    d. Call an ambulance immediately

40. Under what conditions is it advisable to apply a tourniquet to a bleeding body part?
    a. When treating a bleeding pregnant woman
    b. To stop minor bleeding
    c. For any type of bleeding
    d. If the condition is severe

41. Which of the following can you give a conscious patient to keep him/her warm?
    a. Warm liquid, such as hot tea or hot soup
    b. Alcohol-containing beverage
    c. Hot food
    d. Any type of beverage

42. What is an asthmatic attack?
    a. A medical condition common to elderly people
    b. A medical condition that triggers excessive swelling and fever
    c. A medical condition characterized by the swelling of the lining of the bronchial tubes
    d. Heart failure

43. Which of the following are not symptoms of an insect bite?
    a. Breathing difficulties and abdominal cramps
    b. Swelling of the face and lips
    c. Sweating and defecating
    d. Abdominal cramps and increased appetite

44. Seizures can easily be identified by which of the following symptoms?
    a. Convulsions, muscle contractions, loss of apetite and loss of sensation
    b. Fidgeting, confusion and convulsions
    c. Clouded awareness, lip smacking and confusion
    d. All of the above

45. What are the common symptoms of sprains?
    a. Pain in the joint or muscle
    b. Redness and warmth in the injured area
    c. Bruising and swelling in the affected area
    d. Redness and swelling of the affected area

46. What does RICE stand for?
    a. Rest, Ice, Compression and Elevation
    b. Rest, Ice, Compression and Electrolyte
    c. Restructure, Interference, Compression and Electrolyte
    d. Rudiment, Intact, Compression and Elevation

47. Why should you avoid moving an injured person?
    a. You may be unable to lift them properly
    b. You may need some support to lift their weight
    c. In order to avoid exacerbating an injury
    d. None of the above

48. Why should you ask yourself if you can be of help in an emergency situation?
    a. It is a measure of your ability
    b. To ensure that you have the necessary skills to render valuable assistance
    c. It is a rhetorical question with zero impact on your ability
    d. It is routine

49. Under what conditions do you need an extra pair of hands while helping out during an emergency?
    a. If you notice signs of infection
    b. If an injured person feels severe pain
    c. If the injured person feels numbness in the injured area
    d. All of the above

50. What factor determines your response to an accident?
    a. The number of people involved in the accident
    b. The type of vehicle involved in the accident
    c. The type of accident
    d. The available treatment options and first aid equipment

51. What CPR tempo is recommended for a victim of cardiac arrest?
    a. Between 50 and 70 pushes per minute
    b. Between 50 and 80 pushes per minute
    c. Between 100 and 120 pushes per minute
    d. Between 100 and 150 pushes per minute

52. Putting any object in the mouth of a seizure victim is:
    a. A great way to prevent a person from convulsing
    b. An effective way to protect internal organs from collapsing
    c. A recommended solution to any form of seizure
    d. Not recommended under any condition

53. Which of the following is an effective pain reliever for someone bitten or stung by an insect?
    a. Using some painkillers and antibiotics
    b. Applying a disinfectant to the affected area
    c. Applying a paste of baking soda and water to the affected area
    d. Massaging the affected area with a balm

54. How can you assist an asthmatic patient?
    a. Sit the person up
    b. Try to stabilize the victim
    c. Both A and B
    d. None of the above

55. If the asthmatic patient does not have a personal inhaler, what are the available options?
    a. Borrow one
    b. Check the first aid kit
    c. Use an oxygen tank
    d. Do nothing

56. How do you prevent choking in a poison victim?
    a. Give the person a solution of water and laxative drugs
    b. Give the victim a solution of purgatives and laxatives
    c. Turn the person on his/her side
    d. Sit the person up and place his/her head on an elevated object

57. When is it advisable to start CPR?
    a. When the patient is unsteady
    b. When the patient is conscious enough to respond to the CPR
    c. When the patient shows no sign of life
    d. None of the above

58. When applying pressure on a wound with a clean cloth, what do you do if blood soaks through the cloth?
    a. Replace the cloth immediately with a new one
    b. Keep the cloth on the affected area
    c. Put another cloth on the affected area without removing the soaked one
    d. Replace the soaked cloth with a bandage

59. What are common signs of choking?
    a. Loss of consciousness and noisy/difficulty in breathing
    b. Talking difficulty and high temperature
    c. Speech impairment and high temperature
    d. Convulsion and fever

60. A first aid kit should contain all of the following except:
    a. Adhesive tape and different sizes of Band-Aids
    b. A pair of scissors and safety pins of different sizes
    c. Allergy medications and oral decongestants
    d. Disposable sterile gloves, a pair of scissors and syringes

61. What is vaginal route?
    a. A part of the female reproductive system used for childbearing
    b. A part of the female reproductive system used for sexual intercourse
    c. Administration of medications vaginally
    d. The elimination of drugs vaginally

62. Define subcutaneous route.
    a. Drug administration through the skin
    b. Drug administration through injection
    c. Drug administration through blood transfusion
    d. Drug administration through the veins

63. What does Section 5 of the *Physicians' Desk Reference* provide some information on?
    a. Drug dosage and recommended age of users
    b. Drug dosage and potential side effects
    c. Potential side effects and year of production
    d. Name of manufacturer and official website

64. The drugs listed in the *Physicians' Desk Reference* are approved by which of the following?
    a. United States Medical Association
    b. United States Pharmacology Association
    c. Centers for Disease Control
    d. Food and Drug Administration

65. Which groups are at higher risk of adverse drug reactions?
   a. Infants and young children
   b. Infants, young children and nursing mothers
   c. Infants, young children and pregnant women
   d. Infants, young children and the elderly

66. Which of the following does not determine the severity of an adverse drug reaction?
   a. Certain ailments and diseases
   b. Drug factors and heredity
   c. Age and status
   d. None of the above

67. Adverse drug reactions are classified into which of the following?
   a. Dose-related reactions, allergic reactions and idiosyncratic reactions
   b. Idiosyncratic reactions, allergic reactions and impulse reactions
   c. Dose-related reactions, idiosyncratic reactions and reactive reactions
   d. Allergic reactions, dose-related reactions and contributive reactions

68. What is a good drug storage environment?
   a. Humidity-free and have sufficient lighting
   b. Only indirectly exposed to sunlight
   c. Clean and have the desired temperature
   d. All of the above

69. What are the benefits of proper medication storage?
   a. It prevents infestation of pests and vermin
   b. It prevents the usage of contaminated or ineffective drugs
   c. It prevents drug deterioration
   d. All of the above

70. Medications can be damaged by several factors such as:
   a. Heat and moisture
   b. Heat and atmospheric pressure
   c. Moisture and existing climate conditions
   d. Heat and climate conditions

71. What is a result of overdosing on opioids?
    a. Impairment of major body organs
    b. Respiratory depression
    c. Severe kidney and heart problems
    d. Loss of appetite

72. What is the impact of cannabis on a schizophrenia patient?
    a. The medicinal value will improve the patient's condition
    b. It can alleviate the pain associated with the condition
    c. It can worsen the condition
    d. It can trigger other medical conditions

73. Non-medical marijuana may have all of the following effects on users except:
    a. Feelings of relaxation
    b. Reduced blood pressure
    c. Increased appetite
    d. Lower inhibition

74. Cannabis is a derivative of which of the following?
    a. Cannabis marij plant
    b. Cannabis vidic plant
    c. Cannabis sativa plant
    d. Cannabis serum plant

75. Differentiate between psilocybin and mescaline.
    a. Psilocybin is a natural substance found in hallucinogenic mushrooms, while mescaline is found in the mescus cactus
    b. Psilocybin is a natural substance found in hallucinogenic mushrooms, while mescaline is found in the mescus papyrus
    c. Psilocybin is a natural substance found in hallucinogenic mushrooms, while mescaline is found in the peyote cactus
    d. Psilocybin is a natural substance found in hallucinogenic mushrooms, while mescaline is found in the papyrus cactus

76. Define an inhalant.
    a. General name for substances that are inhaled for their medicinal values
    b. General name for substances that are inhaled for their psychoactive effects
    c. General name for substances that are inhaled to increase sexual libido
    d. General name for substances that are inhaled to correct anomalies in the male reproductive system

77. Which of the following are side effects of stimulants?
    a. Developing feelings of hostility and paranoia
    b. Irregular heartbeat and high body temperature
    c. None of the above
    d. All of the above

78. Which of the following side effects of stimulants can lead to addiction?
    a. Short-term effects
    b. Long-term effects
    c. Exhaustion effect
    d. Depression effect

79. While depressants are known for their side effects, what are some medical conditions they can treat?
    a. Social phobia and depression
    b. Insomnia and fever
    c. Panic disorder and irritation
    d. Seizures and high blood pressure

80. What are test protocols?
    a. A set of instructions that must be strictly followed when carrying out laboratory tests
    b. A set of instructions that must be strictly followed when collecting specimens for laboratory analysis
    c. A collection of test cases used to check a specific part of a system
    d. A collection of test cases used to determine the effectiveness of a medical treatment

81. What is the potential effect of a contaminated specimen on a patient?
    a. A wrong diagnosis may lead to complications or loss of life
    b. A contaminated specimen can increase the cost of the test
    c. A contaminated specimen will not have a significant effect on the patient
    d. The impact depends on the type of contaminant and the degree of contamination

82. Some underlying conditions that a sputum test can reveal include all of the following except:
    a. Cystic fibrosis and tuberculosis
    b. Lung abscess and pneumonia
    c. Bronchitis and pneumonia
    d. Lung abscess and jaundice

83. What is the best urine for the timed 24-hour collection?
    a. Urine collected within a 24-hour time frame with the exception of the specimen collected at noon
    b. Urine collected within a 24-hour time frame with the exception of the specimen collected at the 24-hour mark
    c. Urine collected within a 24-hour time frame with the exception of the one collected at the 18-hour mark
    d. All urine collected within a 24-hour time frame

84. Which urine-collection technique guarantees the most reliable test results?
    a. Catheter collection specimen
    b. Midstream clean catch
    c. Timed 24-hour collection
    d. Random specimen

85. Random specimen is the most appropriate specimen collection technique for which of the following?
    a. Urinalysis and microscopic analysis
    b. Urinalysis and pregnancy tests
    c. Tests for respiratory system problems and microscopic analysis
    d. Microscopic analysis and tests for infection of the urinary tract

86. What is a dermal puncture?

a. A procedure for collecting blood from the capillaries
b. A procedure for collecting sputum from tuberculosis patients
c. A procedure for collecting sputum from pregnant women
d. A procedure for collecting blood from pregnant women

87. Which of the following can be used to disinfect a venipuncture site before taking a blood sample?

a. Alcohol and povidone iodine
b. Povidone iodine and methylated spirits
c. Methylated spirits and alcohol
d. Povidone iodine and concentrated methylated spirits

88. In the absence of signs of visible contamination, what is the best solution for cleaning your hands?

a. Water and soap
b. Soap and disinfectant.
c. Alcohol-based hand sanitizer
d. Soap and hand sanitizer

89. Which of the following types of equipment are used for venipunctures?

a. Disposal unit, gloves and tube additives
b. Bandages, gloves and syringes
c. Tourniquet, gloves and face masks
d. Wipes, evacuated tubes and measuring disks

90. Which of the following types of equipment is ideal for collecting multiple blood samples?

a. Evacuated tubes only
b. Evacuated tubes with a tube holder
c. Evacuated tubes with hand gloves
d. Evacuated tubes with measuring cylinders

91. Used items without bloodstains are best discarded in which of the following?

a. Sharps container
b. Leak-proof container
c. Puncture-resistant container
d. General waste container

92. What are some specimens commonly collected for laboratory analysis?
    a. Urine, sputum and saliva
    b. Saliva, sputum and stool
    c. Stool, sputum and urine
    d. Sputum, stool and ear wax

93. Define rumination disorders.
    a. A medical condition characterized by improper digestion
    b. An eating disorder characterized by chewing, regurgitating and rechewing the regurgitated food
    c. A medical condition that results in an inability to chew food properly
    d. A medical condition common to the elderly that prevents them from chewing solid foods

94. What are common symptoms of anorexia nervosa?
    a. Restricted eating patterns and unjustified fear of weight gain
    b. Being considerably underweight and loss of appetite
    c. Living in denial of being underweight and consuming too much water
    d. Inability to eat properly due to health problems

95. What should individuals who are lactose intolerant remove from their diet?
    a. Sauces, canned tuna and beer
    b. Gravy, sweeteners and oily food
    c. Beer, sauces and oranges
    d. Citrus fruits, cabbage and sweeteners

96. Which of the following dietary instructions are great for cancer patients?
    a. Drinking plenty of water and eating carb-rich foods
    b. Drinking plenty of water and eating protein-rich foods
    c. Staying hydrated and eating protein-rich foods
    d. Eating only oily foods and water

97. Excessive salt or sodium consumption can increase an individual's risk of which of the following?

   a. Cancer
   b. High blood pressure
   c. Poor water retention
   d. Respiratory tract infection

98. Hypertensive people should increase their consumption of foods such as:

   a. Whole grains, poultry and low-fat/fat-free products
   b. Sugar-containing drinks, fish and red meats
   c. Lean red meats, poultry and added sugars
   d. Poultry, whole grains and lean red meats

99. Why are whole grains recommended for weight loss?

   a. They are rich in water and other weight-loss components
   b. They are rich in fiber and protein
   c. They are tasty and will encourage healthy eating
   d. They are not expensive and are easy to prepare

100. Why are leafy greens great for weight loss?

   a. They are low in calories and rich in protein content
   b. They are low in calories and rich in essential elements
   c. They have low protein and high fiber content
   d. None of the above

Practice Test 5 – Answers

1) **a:** Six

Food is classified into six classes: proteins, vitamins, carbohydrates, minerals, fats and oils, and water.

2) **a:** Sugars, starches and fiber

Carbohydrates are a class of food whose molecules consist of oxygen, carbon and hydrogen atoms. Dietary carbohydrates are classified into starches, sugars and fiber. They are abundant in nature.

3) **c:** Fish, eggs and meat

Fish, eggs and meat are rich in protein. Soy, beans, some grains and nuts also contain a significant amount of protein.

4) **a:** Fats with high amounts of hydrogen atoms

Saturated fats have high amounts of hydrogen atoms. Processed meats, some plant oils, some pre-packaged snacks and poultry products are some examples of saturated fats.

5) **a:** Oysters, sunflower seeds and salmon

Polyunsaturated fats are fats with more than a single bond. Sunflower oil, safflower oil and corn oil represent the polyunsaturated class. Others are sunflower seeds, oysters and fatty fish such as tuna sardines, mackerel, salmon, herring and trout.

6) **a:** Vitamin C, vitamin B3 and vitamin B12

Water-soluble vitamins do not stay for long in the body because the body cannot store them. As a result, they are passed through urine. Thus, the body needs to replace them more frequently than fat-soluble vitamins. Vitamin C, vitamin B3 and vitamin B12 are examples.

7) **c:** Ulcers, pellagra and beriberi

Beriberi, pellagra and ulcers are some of the medical conditions that are caused by vitamin deficiency. Mouth ulcers, bleeding gums, poor night vision, scaly patches, hair loss and dandruff are other symptoms of a vitamin deficiency.

8) **d:** White rice and white bread

Consuming protein-rich foods and leafy greens, such as beans and legumes, is helpful for weight loss. Conversely, white bread, white rice and other foods rich in carbohydrates can lead to weight gain.

9) **b:** High blood pressure

High blood pressure is a medical condition that can result in a stroke. High blood pressure is otherwise known as hypertension.

10) **c:** They lose their appetite

Cancer patients are prone to malnutrition, thanks to their loss of appetite, taste and smell occasioned by the medical condition or its treatment.

11) **d:** A type of sugar found in animal milk

Lactose is a type of sugar that is commonly found in animal milk. It is also common in dairy products, such as cheese, goat's milk, ice cream and yogurt. Lactose is broken down in the body by lactase, an enzyme.

12) **a:** A disorder characterized by an unusual appetite

Binge-eating disorder is one of the most common eating disorders in young adults and adolescents. People who binge-eat consume large amounts of food within a short period of time. They find it difficult to control their unhealthy eating habits.

13) **b:** The process of collecting tissues or fluids for laboratory analysis

Specimen collection refers to the process through which medical practitioners obtain fluids or tissue for laboratory analysis. Stool, urine and sputum are some specimens that are frequently collected for analysis.

14) **b:** It guarantees accurate diagnosis and treatment

Proper specimen collection is beneficial not only to the provider but to the patient as well. It guarantees accurate diagnosis and treatment and reduces the risk of exposure to pathogens.

15) **c:** Dermal puncture and venipuncture

Dermal punctures and venipunctures are two blood-taking techniques. They require different methods and are designed for different analyses.

16) **d:** A urine specimen that can be taken at any time of the day

Urine specimens can be taken at different times. Random specimen refers to urine specimens collected without time restriction. Thus, such specimens can be taken at any time of the day. It is the easiest and most popular of urine specimens.

17) **b:** Breathing difficulties and coughing

Sputum tests are done for a wide range of reasons. They are ideal for medical conditions that result in coughing and breathing difficulties. The test enables the physician to identify the major cause of the problem through the sputum analysis.

18) **b:** Laboratory quality control

Analytical errors are detected in the laboratory through laboratory quality control. The control process guarantees accurate test results that enable medical health-care providers to provide patients with the best care.

19) **b:** Pharmacology

The branch of science that deals with the study of drugs and their effects on consumers is pharmacology. It covers classes of drugs, drug storage methods and adverse drug reactions, among others.

20) **b:** Five

Drugs are classified into opioids, hallucinogens, inhalants, stimulants and depressants. The classification is based on their attributes, effects and adverse effects on consumers.

21) **c:** Drugs that affect the central nervous system

Depressants affect the central nervous system. This leads to relaxation, sleep, drowsiness and decreased inhibition. In cases of overdose, this can lead to death and coma.

22) **c:** Both A and B

Depressants can have either a temporary or permanent effect on users. Some long-term effects are chronic fatigue, high body temperature, chronic breathing difficulties and sexual problems. Other potential permanent effects are high blood sugar, weight gain, hallucinations, depression and convulsions.

23) **a:** Exhaustion and depression

Stimulants can also have a short-term effect. Exhaustion, depression and apathy are temporary side effects.

24) **b:** They are used as inhalants

Aerosols are used as inhalants. Domestic inhalants include hair sprays, spray paints, deodorant sprays, vegetable oil sprays and aerosol cleaning products for computers.

25) **a:** Lack of coordination and distorted speech

Two short-term effects of inhalants are distorted speech and coordination. Dizziness and euphoria are other temporary effects users can experience, though the effects may also be permanent.

26) **c:** A group of drugs that cause anomalies and changes in consciousness

Hallucinogens may cause perceptual anomalies, hallucinations and changes in the user's emotions, thoughts and consciousness. Some hallucinogens are human-made, while mushrooms and plants are the sources of others.

27) **a:** Psilocybin and mescaline

Two common hallucinogens are mescaline and psilocybin. Other common examples of hallucinogens are PCP, ayahuasca and DMT (dimethyltryptamine). Hallucinogens are otherwise known as dissociative drugs.

28) **d:** None of the above

Regular cannabis use can trigger medical conditions such as selective impairment of cognitive functions, reduction in birth weight, worsening health conditions in schizophrenic patients and impairment of some body organs.

29) **c:** Cannabis is a mood-altering drug, while opioids relieve pain in the nervous system

The major difference between two classes of drugs is that while cannabis is renowned for its mood-altering effects on users, opioids are used for relieving pain in the nervous system.

30) **c:** Storage instructions from the manufacturer

There are several factors to be considered when choosing the most appropriate storage method for a drug. However, none of the factors surpasses the importance of following the manufacturer's storage instructions.

31) **a:** Between 2 and 8°C

Drugs are stored at different temperatures depending on the recommended storage instructions. For instance, for refrigerated medication, the ideal temperature is between 2 and 8°C, while other storage temperatures are determined by the manufacturers' instructions.

32) **a:** They should be stored in a dry, cool place and away from children

While there are specific storage instructions for any type of drug, some general storage conditions apply to all drugs, regardless of the manufacturer or drug type. People are usually advised to store drugs in a dry, cool place, away from children.

33) **c:** Adverse drug reactions

Adverse drug reactions refer to dangerous, unexpected and unwanted reactions to a drug. An adverse drug reaction (ADR) is also referred to as an adverse drug event (ADE) or adverse event.

34) **c:** Severe adverse drug reaction

Death, congenital abnormalities and disabilities are some of the consequences of severe adverse drug reactions. Spina bifida, cerebral palsy, cystic fibrosis, Down syndrome and some heart conditions are some congenital disorders that may be triggered by a severe adverse reaction.

35) **d:** It is a special annual reference guide for physicians

The *Physicians' Desk Reference* is an annually published reference guide for physicians. The voluminous book is a list of all the licensed drugs across the United States. These drugs are approved by the Food and Drug Administration, and the information is published with the assistance of pharmaceutical companies.

36) **d:** All of the above

Some information you can find in the *Physicians' Desk Reference* includes controlled substance categories, contact information for state DEA programs, drug dosage and drug indications.

37) **a:** Manufacturer's address and page numbers of where you can find additional information on specific subjects

The *Physicians' Desk Reference* is divided into six sections. Section 2 contains information such as manufacturer's address and page numbers of where you can find additional information on specific subjects.

38) **b:** The initial medical assistance provided to a patient before the arrival of higher-level medical care

First aid is the first form of treatment offered to someone suffering from a sudden ailment or injury. The objective is to prevent the situation from deteriorating until competent medical staff is on hand to attend to the medical condition.

39) **b:** Apply pressure to the affected area with a clean cloth

To stop bleeding, use a clean cloth to apply direct pressure on the source of the wound that leads to the bleeding. Alternatively, use a piece of gauze or tissue until the bleeding stops.

40) **d:** If the condition is severe

Using a tourniquet is not recommended. However, under some conditions, such as severe bleeding, a tourniquet may be applied to get the bleeding under control.

41) **a:** Warm liquid, such as hot tea or hot soup

You can give someone suffering from cold exposure hot tea or hot soup to increase their body temperature. However, refrain from offering beverages containing alcohol. Alcohol-based beverages can complicate issues, especially if the patient is suffering from hypothermia.

42) **c:** A medical condition characterized by the swelling of the lining of the bronchial tubes

Asthma is a chronic disease characterized by the inflammation and swelling of the bronchial tubes' lining. It usually causes difficulty in breathing and may lead to sudden death if the patient is not attended to promptly.

43) **a:** Breathing difficulties and abdominal cramps

Insect bites or stings can come with some painful symptoms. Notable symptoms are swelling of the face and lips. Sweating is also a common symptom. Increased appetite and abdominal cramps are other symptoms.

44) **d:** All of the above

Seizures are identified by symptoms such as loss of appetite and loss of sensation. Clouded awareness, muscle contractions, lip smacking and fidgeting are some other symptoms.

45) **d:** Redness and swelling of the affected area

Sprains occur when the ligament's fibers are partially or completely torn. Someone may experience a knee, wrist, ankle or thumb sprain, although ankle sprains are the most common. Redness and swelling of the affected area are common signs of sprains.

46) **a:** Rest, Ice, Compression and Elevation

The RICE approach is one of the most recommended methods for treating sprains. The acronym stands for Rest, Ice, Compression and Elevation. This refers to each step that must be taken to treat the victim.

47) **c:** In order to avoid exacerbating an injury

Moving an injured person is problematic because you may not be able to see things like internal bleeding and fractures. Moving a person with these injuries could worsen the problem.

48) **b:** To ensure that you have the necessary skills to render valuable assistance

When you are faced with an emergency situation and feel compelled to render assistance, it is imperative that you first ask yourself if you can be of help. Do you have the skills needed to render assistance, or will you end up wasting your time and that of the patient?

49) **d:** All of the above

While helping out during an emergency, you may call for backup if you notice signs of infection, if the injured person is uncomfortable and feels severe pain or if the person feels numbness in the affected area.

50) **c:** The type of accident

Your response to an accident should be determined by the nature of the accident. Your response to a fire will be different from your response to a flood. Hence, it is imperative that you know the type of accident to be able to determine the approach to use.

51) **c:** Between 100 and 120 pushes per minute

A victim of cardiac arrest will experience breathing difficulties. To keep the patient alive, CPR of between 100 and 120 pushes per minute is recommended. This tempo gives the chest enough room to return to its normal position before the next push.

52) **d:** Not recommended under any condition

Putting any object in the mouth of a seizure victim is erroneously considered by many as an effective first aid measure. However, it is not a recommended treatment for seizures and can cause the patient great harm.

53) **c:** Applying a paste of baking soda and water to the affected area

Aside from applying pressure to the affected area with a clean cloth, applying a paste of baking soda and water on the affected area is also an effective pain reliever for someone stung or bitten by an insect.

54) **c:** Both A and B

Asthmatic patients can die if they are not quickly treated. To assist a person having an asthma attack, sit the person up and try to stabilize him/her. Loosen any tight clothing around the neck to facilitate breathing.

55) **b:** Check the first aid kit

If the asthmatic patient does not have a personal inhaler, do not borrow an inhaler from a random person. Rather, check the first aid kit for an inhaler.

56) **c:** Turn the person on his/her side

To prevent a poison victim from choking, turn him/her to the side. Administering a solution of laxative drugs and water or offering a purgative will be of no help.

57) **c:** When the patient shows no sign of life

If a patient is showing no signs of life, you should start CPR immediately.

58) **c:** Put another cloth on the affected area without removing the soaked one

When applying pressure on a wound with a clean cloth, if the cloth is soaked in blood, do not remove the first cloth. Apply another cloth on top of the one you already used and continue applying pressure.

59) **a:** Loss of consciousness and noisy/difficulty in breathing

An adult or a young child can experience choking when a foreign object lodges in the victim's windpipe or throat and blocks airflow. The blockage can be life-threatening. Choking is identified by noisy breathing, breathing difficulty or loss of consciousness.

60) **d:** Disposable sterile gloves, a pair of scissors and syringes

A first aid kit comes with the necessary tools for rendering first aid during emergencies. A first aid kit should contain disposable sterile gloves, a pair of scissors, adhesive tape and safety pins of different sizes. It generally will not contain syringes.

61) **c:** Administration of medications vaginally

Drugs are administered to patients via different routes. Vaginal route refers to drugs or medications administration vaginally. Women may absorb drugs administered as a tablet, solution, ring or gel through their vaginal walls.

62) **b:** Drug administration through injection

This is a form of drug administration through injection. A needle is inserted beneath the skin to inject the drug. The drug moves into the capillaries or small blood vessels on its way to the bloodstream.

63) **b:** Drug dosage and potential side effects

Section 5 of the *Physicians' Desk Reference* provides information about drug dosage and potential side effects of drugs on users.

64) **d:** Food and Drug Administration

The drugs listed in the *Physicians' Desk Reference* are approved by the Food and Drug Administration, proof of the drugs' acceptance by the appropriate regulatory body.

65) **d:** Infants, young children and the elderly

While people of all ages can react adversely to drugs, adverse drug reactions are most common in infants, young children and the elderly. Young children and infants have low metabolisms, while the elderly may have underlying health conditions that may trigger the adverse reaction.

66) **c:** Age and status

The severity of the adverse drug reactions on patients is determined by a long list of factors. This includes diseases, age, drugs, certain ailments and heredity.

67) **a:** Dose-related reactions, allergic reactions and idiosyncratic reactions

Adverse drug reactions are classified into dose-related reactions, idiosyncratic reactions and allergic reactions. The mechanism behind each reaction is the determining factor for the classification.

68) **d:** All of the above

A good storage environment should be clean, have the right temperature, be humidity-free and have sufficient lighting. Direct sunlight may damage the stored drugs.

69) **d:** All of the above

Storing drugs properly prevents infestation of vermin and pests, prevents the use of ineffective or contaminated drugs and prevents drug deterioration.

70) **a:** Heat and moisture

Medications can be damaged by heat and moisture. Direct exposure to sunlight is another factor that may damage or reduce the potency of a drug. Humidity is another destructive factor.

71) **b:** Respiratory depression

Overdosing on any drug can lead to many medical conditions. When someone overdoses on opioids, this can cause respiratory depression, a medical condition that causes slow breathing known as hypoventilation.

72) **c:** It can worsen the condition

Cannabis can affect a user adversely. Schizophrenia patients, especially, should steer clear of using marijuana because it can worsen their condition and make it more difficult to manage the ailment.

73) **d:** Lower inhibition

Non-medical marijuana may have a wide range of effects on users. Some common effects are reduced blood pressure, increased appetite for food, lightheadedness and feelings of relaxation. It does not lower inhibition.

74) **c:** Cannabis sativa plant

Cannabis is made up of over 120 compounds with potentially different properties from the leaves, flowering tops, seeds and stems of the cannabis sativa plant, otherwise known as hemp.

75) **c:** Psilocybin is a natural substance found in hallucinogenic mushrooms, while mescaline is found in the peyote cactus

Psilocybin and mescaline are two common hallucinogens. The former is a natural substance found in hallucinogenic mushrooms, while the latter is found in the peyote cactus. Other examples are LSD or D-lysergic acid diethylamide and dimethyltryptamine (DMT).

76) **b:** General name for substances that are inhaled for their psychoactive effects

An inhalant is a general name for substances that are inhaled to provide mind-altering or psychoactive effects on the user. Some examples of inhalants are aerosol sprays, solvents and nitrites.

77) **d:** All of the above

Stimulants have several side effects. Some common ones are paranoia, high body temperature, irregular heartbeat and unhealthy feelings of hostility. Higher doses may cause anxiety, coma, tension, seizures and death.

78) **c:** Exhaustion effect

Exhaustion is one of the common effects of using stimulants. The exhaustion effect is the reason why most users have an excessive craving for the drug. If the inordinate craving is not controlled, it can lead to addiction over time.

79) **a:** Social phobia and depression

While depressants are known for their side effects, they are used to treat a wide range of medical conditions, such as social phobias and depression. They are also used to treat obsessive compulsive disorder, seizures and insomnia.

80) **c:** A collection of test cases used to check a specific part of a system

Test protocols are a collection of test cases designed to check a specific part of a system. Each of the test cases should contain some important information, such as the purpose of the test, the criteria for acceptance, and requirements that must be met before the test is performed.

81) **a:** A wrong diagnosis may lead to complications or loss of life

A contaminated specimen will give the wrong result. If a patient is misdiagnosed as a result of the contamination, the patient may have to contend with potentially deadly complications.

82) **d:** Lung abscess and jaundice

Some underlying conditions that a sputum test can reveal include bronchitis, cystic fibrosis, pneumonia, tuberculosis, chronic obstructive pulmonary disease and lung abscesses.

83) **d:** All urine collected within a 24-hour time frame

Batches of urine are collected over 24 hours. All urine is collected in a large-collection bottle and is preserved with the addition of a preservative to prevent urinary components from breaking down.

84) **b:** Midstream clean catch

Midstream clean catch is the urine-collection technique that guarantees the most reliable test result. Before the specimen-taking process, the patient must first use a castile soap towelette to cleanse the urethral area. Then, the first portion of the urine is voided as a preventive measure against obtaining contaminated urine.

85) **a:** Urinalysis and microscopic analysis

For urinalysis and microscopic analysis, the random specimen technique is the most appropriate for specimen collection. Random specimen refers to a urine specimen that can be taken at any time of the day. Due to the ease of taking the specimen, it remains the most commonly used form of specimen.

86) **a:** A procedure for collecting blood from the capillaries

An effective blood-collecting technique for laboratory analysis is a dermal puncture. This procedure is used for collecting blood from capillaries. Since capillaries are between veins and arteries, the blood collected through this technique is a mixture of blood from the arteries and veins.

87) **a:** Alcohol and povidone iodine

Before taking a blood sample, the target site must be disinfected first. You have two options to choose from to do this: using alcohol as the disinfectant or using povidone iodine. However, the iodine solution is less effective than alcohol.

88) **c:** Alcohol-based hand sanitizer

In the absence of signs of visible contamination, the best solution for keeping your hands clean is using alcohol-based hand sanitizer. If your hands are contaminated, wash them with water and soap.

89) **a:** Disposal unit, gloves and tube additives

Several types of equipment are used for venipunctures. These include gloves, disposal units and tube additives. Others are gauze, collection or evacuated tubes, needles, wipes or swabs, tourniquets and gloves.

90) **b:** Evacuated tubes with a tube holder

For multiple blood collection, use evacuated tubes with a tube holder and a needle to enable you to fill the tubes directly. Before filling the tube, place it into a rack. Alternatively, use a winged needle set or a syringe for the same purpose.

91) **d:** General waste container

Items with bloodstains are discarded in special containers designed for that purpose. However, those without bloodstains should be discarded in a general waste container since they pose no risk of infecting people through blood-borne pathogens.

92) **c:** Stool, sputum and urine

Stool, urine and sputum are some specimens that are frequently collected for analysis.

93) **b:** An eating disorder characterized by chewing, regurgitating and rechewing the regurgitated food

Rumination disorder refers to an eating disorder in which the victim regurgitates previously chewed food, re-chews the food, re-swallows it or spits it out. This eating disorder can develop in infancy, childhood or adulthood.

94) **a:** Restricted eating patterns and unjustified fear of weight gain

Some common symptoms of anorexia nervosa are restricted eating patterns and unjustified fear of weight gain.

95) **a:** Sauces, canned tuna and beer

People who are lactose intolerant should remove lactose-containing foods from their diet. They should not consume canned tuna, sauces, gravy, sweeteners and beer. These foods are rich in lactose and may trigger negative reactions.

96) **c:** Staying hydrated and eating protein-rich foods

Cancer patients are advised to eat lots of fruits. They should also increase their protein consumption to allow their body to repair the damaging side effects that may arise from treating the ailment.

97) **b:** High blood pressure

Excessive sodium consumption can increase a consumer's risk of high blood pressure. This is due to the ability of the salt or sodium to increase the body's fluid retention, thus triggering increased blood pressure.

98) **a:** Whole grains, poultry and low-fat/fat-free products

Hypertensive people can manage their condition well if they choose their foods wisely. It is best that they include foods that are low in cholesterol, saturated fat, added sugars and salt. They should also eat more foods that are rich in protein, nutrients and fiber.

99) **b:** They are rich in fiber and protein

Whole grains are recommended for weight loss because they are loaded with protein and fiber. Some whole grains, such as oats, also possess soluble fiber that improves metabolic health and ensures satiety.

100) **a:** They are low in calories and rich in protein content

Leafy greens, such as spinach, Swiss chard and kale, are low in carbohydrates and calories, making them perfect for weight loss. They are also rich in fiber, another important weight-loss attribute.

Practice Test 6

1. What are carbohydrates?
    a. A class of food whose molecules consist of carbon, hydrogen and oxygen atoms
    b. A class of food whose molecules consist of carbon, fluorine and oxygen atoms
    c. A class of food whose molecules consist of carbon, sulfur and oxygen atoms
    d. A class of food whose molecules consist of carbon, hydrogen and ozone

2. Which of the following are not healthy carbohydrates?
    a. Vegetables, tubers and nuts
    b. Fruits, whole grains and white bread
    c. Whole fruits, whole grains and legumes
    d. Seeds, vegetables and nuts

3. Which of the following are not bad carbohydrates?
    a. Ice cream, fruit juices and sugary drinks
    b. Sugary drinks, fruit juices and cookies
    c. Cookies, pastries and fruit juices
    d. Seeds, tubers and vegetables

4. Protein makes up how much of an average person's total body weight?
    a. 20%
    b. 16%
    c. 50%
    d. 36%

5. How does the human body get the recommended amount of amino acids?
    a. It naturally produces the amount it needs
    b. It produces half of the needed quantity, while the rest is obtained from food
    c. It modifies other amino acids
    d. Amino acid supplements are the main source of amino acids

6. Fats should make up less than how much of your calories?
    a. 30% of your daily calories
    b. 50% of your monthly calories
    c. 40% of your weekly calories
    d. 20% of your annual calories

7. Fats are classified into:
    a. Simple fats and complex fats
    b. Primary fats and secondary fats
    c. Saturated fats unsaturated fats
    d. Amino acid fats and fiber fats

8. Define macro-minerals.
    a. Mineral elements that the body needs in large quantities to enable some organs to perform their functions properly
    b. Mineral elements that the body needs in small quantities to enable some organs to perform their functions properly
    c. Mineral elements that the body needs under special medical conditions to enable some organs to perform their functions properly
    d. Mineral elements that the elderly need to enable some of their body organs to perform their functions properly

9. What are some examples of trace minerals?
    a. Zinc, fluoride and iron
    b. Iron, iodine and chloride
    c. Calcium, cobalt and potassium
    d. Sulfur, fluoride and zinc

10. Water serves which of the following purposes?
    a. Toxin removal and dehydration prevention
    b. Nutrient transportation and lubricating body organs
    c. Constipation prevention and urinary tract infection prevention
    d. All of the above

11. What is the primary benefit of weight control?
    a. To look more attractive
    b. To enable you to wear trendy clothes
    c. To prevent body shaming
    d. To be in shape and stay healthy

12. Which of the following weight-control components can be found in whole grains?
    a. Soluble fiber and protein
    b. Carbohydrates and soluble fiber
    c. Fats and soluble fiber
    d. Carbohydrates and protein

13. Although fruits are sugary, why are they considered healthy carbohydrates?
    a. Because they are a natural source of energy
    b. Because they are less expensive than artificial sugar
    c. Because they have low energy density
    d. Because they have high energy density

14. Hypertensive patients should stay away from foods that are rich in which of the following?
    a. Nutrients, protein and fiber
    b. Saturated fat, protein and fiber
    c. Added sugars, proteins and nutrients
    d. Salt, protein and fiber

15. What is lactose sensitivity?
    a. A lack of sufficient lactase to break down and digest lactose
    b. A lack of sufficient lactose to break down and digest lactase
    c. A lack of sufficient fructose to break down and digest fructase
    d. A lack of sufficient fructase to break down and digest fructose

16. Why are lactose-free products healthy for people who are sensitive to lactose?
    a. They contain enough lactase to break the lactose down
    b. They are special types of foods with minimal or zero lactose
    c. They contain the right amount of enzymes to neutralize the effect of lactose
    d. They are canned lactose-free foods

17. What are eating disorders?
    a. Eating behaviors peculiar to newborn babies
    b. A condition wherein a person is unable to consume the right amount of food
    c. Medical conditions that lead to overeating and overdrinking
    d. Medical conditions that can affect the patient emotionally and health-wise

18. What triggers eating disorders?
    a. Food scarcity
    b. High appetite
    c. Unusual obsession with food
    d. Unusual obsession with one's weight

19. Define anorexia nervosa.
    a. An eating disorder characterized by excessive eating of fatty foods
    b. An eating disorder characterized by excessive consumption of junk food
    c. An eating disorder common to people who always consider themselves overweight
    d. An eating disorder common to people who always consider themselves underweight

20. What is rumination disorder?
    a. An eating disorder common to infants and the elderly
    b. An eating disorder common to people irrespective of their age
    c. An eating disorder common to people who live a sedentary lifestyle
    d. An eating disorder that leads to dehydration and loss of appetite

21. What must you do before applying a tourniquet?
    a. Apply methylated alcohol on the area where a tourniquet is to be applied
    b. Look for an artery to use
    c. Look for an appropriate and visible vein
    d. None of the above

22. The best disinfectant for a venipuncture site is which of the following?
    a. 50% alcohol swab
    b. 70% alcohol swab
    c. 30% alcohol swab
    d. 60% alcohol swab

23. What is a major difference between a dermal puncture and venipuncture?
    a. A dermal puncture requires more precision than a venipuncture
    b. A dermal puncture is more expensive than a venipuncture
    c. A venipuncture is for special medical conditions, while a dermal puncture is for taking blood specimens for a wide range of medical conditions.
    d. A dermal puncture requires less precision than a venipuncture

24. What is the major side effect of a dermal puncture?
    a. It takes a longer processing time than a venipuncture
    b. It is more expensive than a venipuncture
    c. It is less desirable than a venipuncture
    d. The process is faster than a venipuncture

25. What are factors that determine the type of information that can be derived from urine tests?
    a. The collection technique and timing
    b. The collection technique and density of the urine
    c. The collection technique and the type of test done
    d. The collection technique and the reagents used

26. Which collection technique produces concentrated urine?
    a. Last morning specimen
    b. First morning specimen
    c. Random specimen
    d. Midstream clean catch

27. What is another name for a first morning specimen?
    a. 12-hour specimen
    b. 8-hour specimen
    c. 16-hour specimen
    d. 24-hour specimen

28. Which of the following is not a specimen collection guideline?
    a. Specimens should be transported in glass containers
    b. Collection tubes should be properly labeled
    c. Transporting containers shouldn't be reused
    d. Transporting containers should be free of particles

29. How are drugs classified?
    a. By their chemical activity and physical attributes
    b. By their chemical activity and cost of production
    c. By their chemical activity and conditions treated by the drug
    d. By their physical activity and chemical properties

30. What are barbiturates?
    a. Depressants that affect the respiratory system
    b. Depressants that affect the central nervous system
    c. Special types of inhalants for asthmatic patients
    d. Special inhalants for people with urinary tract infections

31. What are stimulants?
    a. Drugs for treating depression and apathy
    b. Drugs used for treating irritation and apathy
    c. Drugs used to induce vomiting under special conditions
    d. Drugs that can increase a patient's alertness temporarily

32. What are some side effects of stimulants?
    a. Increased alertness and the desire to talk excessively
    b. Increased blood pressure and low heartbeat
    c. Low heartbeat and fever
    d. High body temperature and typhoid

33. Which of the following are examples of nitrites?
    a. Video head cleaner
    b. Leather cleaner
    c. Liquid aroma
    d. All of the above

34. Commercial household gases that are used as inhalants include which of the following?
    a. Whipped cream aerosol and butane lighters
    b. Propane tanks and whipped cream aerosols
    c. Both A and B
    d. None of the above

35. Which of the following are long-term effects of inhalants?
    a. Delayed behavioral development and liver damage
    b. Lack of coordination and euphoria
    c. Kidney damage and slurred speech
    d. Dizziness and lack of coordination

36. Hallucinogens are used for both religious rituals and recreational purposes due to which of the following?
    a. Their ability to change a user's thoughts and emotions
    b. Their popularity among youth
    c. Their ease of purchase and use
    d. Their low cost and ease of use

37. Which of the following is the most popular and most commonly used illegal drug?
    a. Marijuana
    b. Inhalants
    c. Depressants
    d. Hallucinogens

38. Cannabis is made up of:
    a. Over 100 compounds with overlapping properties
    b. Over 120 compounds with distinct properties
    c. Over 50 compounds with some similar and some different properties
    d. Over 150 properties with some similarities and differences

39. Medical marijuana can be used to treat a wide range of ailments that include which of the following?
    a. Sleep disturbances, chronic pain and muscle spasticity
    b. Muscle spasticity, diarrhea and loss of concentration
    c. Diarrhea, high blood pressure and blisters
    d. Diarrhea, fever and low blood pressure

40. What are opioids?
    a. Pain relievers that work on the respiratory system
    b. Pain relievers that work on the urinary system
    c. Pain relievers that work on the nervous system
    d. Pain relievers that work on the reproductive system

41. Medications that are meant to be stored at cool temperatures are best stored which temperatures?
    a. Between 2°C and 8°C
    b. Between 8°C and 15°C
    c. Between 12°C and 18°C
    d. Between 20°C and 25°C

42. What is a dose-related adverse drug reaction?
    a. An adverse drug reaction triggered by overdosing on a drug
    b. An exaggeration of the therapeutic effect of a drug
    c. An adverse drug reaction triggered by overdosing on depressants
    d. An adverse drug reaction triggered by overdosing on inhalants

43. Define idiosyncratic adverse drug reaction.
    a. An adverse drug reaction that is triggered by some special temperature conditions
    b. An adverse drug reaction that is triggered by some special medical conditions
    c. An adverse drug reaction that is triggered by some mechanisms that are not yet understood
    d. An adverse drug reaction that is triggered by an individual's response to drugs

44. How does heredity determine the severity of adverse drug reactions?
    a. Allergies to some drugs may be passed down through the generations
    b. Some people can suddenly develop adverse reactions to some drugs
    c. People whose parents are allergic to some drugs may react adversely
    d. People whose children are allergic to some drugs may develop an immunity to their side effects

45. What is another factor that can influence adverse drug reactions?
    a. Weight and size
    b. Certain diseases and ailments
    c. Existing political and economic situation
    d. None of the above

46. Diagnostic product information can be found where in the *Physicians' Desk Reference*?
    a. Section 3
    b. Section 4
    c. Section 5
    d. Section 6

47. The generic name and brand name of each drug can be found where in the *Physicians' Desk Reference*?
    a. Section 3
    b. Section 4
    c. Section 5
    d. Section 2

48. Which of the following are not drug administration techniques?
    a. Oral administration and subcutaneous route
    b. Subcutaneous route and intramuscular route
    c. Vaginal route and nasal route
    d. Vaginal route and intramuscular route

49. What are some minor injuries that may require first aid?
    a. Nasal congestion and sore throat
    b. Sprains and abrasions
    c. Sore throat and cough
    d. All of the above

50. When does choking occur?
    a. When someone consumes too large a quantity of food within a short time frame
    b. When someone does not have access to regular airflow
    c. When a foreign object lodges in someone's throat
    d. When someone is suddenly hit from the back

51. What are some common signs of choking are?
    a. Difficulty in breathing and talking
    b. Flushed skin and loss of consciousness
    c. Lips and skin turning blue and flushed skin
    d. All of the above

52. Which of the following is one of the ways the windpipe can be cleared of choking?
    a. Slapping the person's back ten times
    b. Standing behind the person and bending him/her at the waist
    c. Both A and B
    d. None of the above

53. To stop bleeding, do the following first:
    a. Wash the surface with methylated spirits
    b. Wrap the affected area with a bandage
    c. Apply pressure to the affected area with a clean cloth
    d. Wash the affected area with soap and water

54. Why is it important to raise the affected area above the heart?
    a. To relieve the pain
    b. To make it easier to assist the patient
    c. To reduce the flow of blood
    d. All of the above

55. You may consider calling a doctor if you are faced with the following condition:
    a. If the patient feels feverish or may be bleeding internally
    b. If the patient is an adult
    c. If the patient is not living in the neighborhood
    d. If the patient is a minor

56. What is hypothermia?
    a. A sudden increase in someone's body temperature
    b. A sudden decrease in someone's body temperature
    c. A sudden increase in someone's blood pressure
    d. A sudden decrease in someone's blood pressure

57. What is the best treatment for a frostbite victim?
    a. Wrapping the affected area with a cloth dipped in hot water
    b. Wrapping the affected area with a soft and loose cloth
    c. Wrapping the affected area with a cloth dipped in methylated spirits
    d. Wrapping the affected area with a cloth dipped in iodine

58. To treat someone with hypothermia, which of the following is advisable?
    a. Warming the arms and legs
    b. Heating the person with a heating lamp or a hot bath
    c. Offering the person alcohol or cigarettes
    d. None of the above

59. What is poisoning?
    a. An injury or death caused by consuming too much food
    b. An injury or death caused by consuming food rich in sugar and salt
    c. An injury or death caused by swallowing harmful gases or drugs
    d. An injury or death caused by drinking too much water

60. Which of the following is a major determinant of the most effective treatment for poisoning?
    a. The quantity of the poison consumed
    b. The type of poison consumed
    c. The strength of the victim's immune system
    d. The victim's weight and height

61. A little boy is poisoned in the eye. What is the best first aid treatment for him?
    a. He should be made to sit up and bend his head
    b. Flush the eye with lukewarm water and disinfectant gently
    c. Flush the eye with lukewarm water
    d. Flush the eye with cold water and disinfectant gently

62. When you call an ambulance for a poisoning case, take the following along:
    a. Pill bottles, the packages or the pill container
    b. The packages, pill container and instruction manual
    c. Everything in the vicinity of the patient
    d. None of the above

63. Inducing vomiting with syrup of ipecac is considered:
    a. A surefire way of curing cases of poisoning
    b. An option that should not be considered due to its high risk
    c. A great option when combined with other treatment options
    d. The easiest treatment for poisoning

64. What is the importance of asking for an asthma plan when assisting an asthmatic patient?
    a. It helps you gather necessary information you will present to the medical team
    b. It enables you to understand the patient's medication
    c. It is a mere routine that must be followed
    d. It has no significant effect on the patient

65. What do you do first when offering first aid to a victim of insect bite or sting?
    a. Wash the affected area with water and soap
    b. Remove an embedded stinger by scraping the surface gently
    c. Place ice on the area for a couple of minutes
    d. Apply a paste of water and baking soda to the affected area

66. Which of the following medications are effective for treating insect bites or stings?
    a. Ibuprofen and paracetamol
    b. Antihistamine tablets and hydrocortisone ointment
    c. Crotamiton lotion and antihistamine tablets
    d. All of the above

67. Which of the following medications are effective for treating headaches?
    a. Acetaminophen
    b. Ibuprofen
    c. Both A and B
    d. None of the above

68. Which of the following is not a way to assist a victim of seizure?
    a. Loosening anything that makes breathing difficult
    b. Not putting anything in the person's mouth
    c. Not restraining the person's movements
    d. Restraining the person's movements

69. What is cardiac arrest?
   a. A medical condition that arises from insufficient blood flow to the heart muscle
   b. A medical condition that refers to loss of heart function, breathing and consciousness
   c. A medical condition that slows down the operations of the heart
   d. A mild medical condition with symptoms such as increased appetite and sweating

70. Differentiate between cardiac arrest and heart attack.
   a. Cardiac arrest is a halting of blood flow to the heart muscle, while heart attack is a loss of breathing and consciousness
   b. Heart attack is a halting of blood flow to the heart muscle, while cardiac arrest is a loss of breathing and consciousness
   c. Cardiac arrest is a halting of blood flow to the heart, while heart attack is a loss of heart cardiac flow
   d. Heart attack is a halting of blood flow to the heart muscle, while cardiac arrest is a loss of the use of major body organs

71. Which part of the RICE approach for treating sprains should be done for two consecutive days?
   a. Rest
   b. Ice
   c. Compression
   d. Elevation

72. When responding to emergencies, you should take all of the following precautions except:
   a. Checking for bleeding
   b. Not moving the injured person
   c. Checking for fractures
   d. Waiting for a physician to perform CPR

73. Define sprains.
   a. The dislocation of major body joints
   b. Ligament injuries caused by torn ligament fibers
   c. Injuries to the limbs
   d. Injuries to the skull caused by a slip or fall

74. Your response to an accident should be determined by which of the following?
    a. The number of accident victims
    b. The seriousness of the accident
    c. The type of accident
    d. None of the above

75. How long do seizures last?
    a. Between two and five minutes
    b. Between one and two minutes
    c. Between 30 seconds and two minutes
    d. Between 30 seconds and one minute

76. Why is massaging not a great way to treat hypothermia?
    a. It is expensive
    b. It is extremely difficult to perform
    c. It may damage the heart and lungs
    d. It requires some special skills

77. Which of these is irrelevant when offering first aid?
    a. Checking the scene for signs of potential danger
    b. Calling for medical assistance if necessary
    c. Providing care immediately.
    d. Waiting for permission from the patient or relatives before rendering assistance

78. What is the primary objective of first aid?
    a. To prevent a health condition from deteriorating
    b. To reduce medical expenses
    c. To have enough evidence of the incident warranting the first aid
    d. None of the above

79. What factors determine the most appropriate drug administration method?
    a. The drug's formula and how it works
    b. The cost of the drug and the part of the body to be treated
    c. The physician's years of experience and the drug's formula
    d. The part of the body to be treated and the cost of treatment

80. Which of the following is a common example of a drug administered through the vaginal route?
    a. Ibuprofen
    b. Ampiclox
    c. Estrogen
    d. Esterogen

81. What parts of the body are commonly used for intramuscular drug administration?
    a. Upper arm and thigh
    b. Thigh and muscles of the chest
    c. Upper arm and lower abdomen
    d. Upper arm and neck muscle

82. What is the safest and most convenient drug administration technique?
    a. Oral administration
    b. Intramuscular administration
    c. Vaginal administration
    d. Subcutaneous administration

83. Where can you easily find drug names and other information in the *Physicians' Desk Reference*?
    a. Section 1
    b. Section 2
    c. Section 3
    d. Section 4

84. The *Physicians' Desk Reference* is a collaborative effort between which of the following?
    a. The medical profession and the Food and Drug Administration
    b. The Food and Drug Administration and pharmaceutical companies
    c. Pharmaceutical companies and medical workers
    d. The Food and Drug Administration and Patients' Welfare Board

85. What are some factors that may increase adverse drug reactions?
    a. Age and hereditary factors
    b. Hereditary factors and weight
    c. Height and certain ailments
    d. Drug factors and height

86. Which of the following are factors that can destroy the efficiency of a drug?
    a. Heat and moisture
    b. Heat and light
    c. Moisture and light
    d. All of the above

87. Why are opioids used for treating moderate pain?
    a. They come into effect within a few hours
    b. They block pain signals between the brain and the body
    c. They act like a placebo
    d. They boost the body's immune system

88. Some common examples of hallucinogens include all of the following except:
    a. Ayahuasca and PCP
    b. Mescaline and psilocybin
    c. Dimethyltryptamine and ayahuasca
    d. None of the above

89. Which of the following is used for spiritual purposes?
    a. Depressants
    b. Inhalants
    c. Hallucinogens
    d. Medical cannabis

90. Which ailments can be treated with depressants?
    a. Insomnia and seizures
    b. Hallucinations and high blood sugar
    c. Chronic breathing difficulties and sexual problems
    d. Sexual problems and high blood sugar

91. What are benzodiazepines?
    a. Psychoactive drugs for treating infections and high blood pressure
    b. Psychoactive drugs for treating anxiety and high blood pressure
    c. Psychoactive drugs for treating infections and anxiety
    d. Psychoactive drugs for treating insomnia and anxiety

92. Barbiturates are which of the following?
    a. Central nervous system depressants
    b. Respiratory system depressants
    c. Urinary system depressants
    d. Reproductive system depressants

93. What are necessary precautions when storing reagents?
    a. Leave them sitting for a long time so they become concentrated
    b. Read and follow storage instructions
    c. Both A and B
    d. None of the above

94. What determines the usability of the result of an analysis?
    a. Time of analysis and years of experience of the analyst
    b. Years of experience of the analyst and the purpose of the analysis
    c. Accuracy and reliability of the result of the analysis
    d. Accuracy and years of experience of the analyst

95. How is urine collected through the timed 24-hour technique preserved?
    a. Through the addition of preservatives or refrigeration
    b. Through the addition of preservatives or iodine solution
    c. Through refrigeration and addition of iodine solution
    d. Through the addition of methylated spirits and iodine solution

96. What is the major shortcoming of the random specimen technique?
    a. It is expensive
    b. It is a time-consuming technique
    c. It provides false and misleading information
    d. It is limited to certain medical conditions

97. What are some shortcomings of the dermal puncture sample collection procedure?
    a. It may result in loss of life
    b. It may increase a patient's medical expenses
    c. It may result in hemolysis or blood clotting
    d. All of the above

98. How can people stay hydrated?
    a. Drinking water only
    b. Drinking water and carbonated drinks
    c. Drinking water and canned juice
    d. Drinking water and freshly squeezed juices

99. What is one of the most important nutrients needed by the body?
    a. Fats and oil
    b. Minerals
    c. Essential elements
    d. Water

100. Which of the following is not a function of water in the body?
    a. It lubricates body organs
    b. It serves as a shock absorber
    c. It removes toxins
    d. It leads to frequent urination

Practice Test 6 – Answers

1) **a:** A class of food whose molecules consist of carbon, hydrogen and oxygen atoms

Carbohydrates are a member of the triune classes of food, collectively known as macronutrients, alongside protein and fat.

2) **b:** Fruits, whole grains and white bread

Carbohydrates are classified according to how healthy they are. Healthy amounts of carbohydrates are present in whole fruits, legumes, whole grains, vegetables, tubers, seeds and nuts.

3) **d:** Seeds, tubers and vegetables

Bad carbohydrates include fruit juices, ice cream, cookies, sugary drinks and pastries. They should be consumed in moderation.

4) **b:** 16%

Protein makes up 16% of a human body and helps ensure healthy bones, muscles, hair, cells and skin.

5) **c:** It modifies other amino acids

While the body can produce only a fraction of the amino acids it needs, it makes up for the inadequacy by modifying other amino acids.

6) **a:** 30% of your daily calories

According to recent research, a healthy diet is incomplete without healthy fats. While it is true that fat contains high calories, the human body needs these calories as a source of energy. The World Health Organization recommends limiting fats to fewer than 30% of one's daily calories.

7) **c:** Saturated fats and unsaturated fats

Fats are classified into saturated fats and unsaturated fats. Saturated fats have high amounts of hydrogen atoms, while unsaturated fats contain double bonds and are liquid at room temperature.

8) **a:** Mineral elements that the body needs in large quantities to enable some organs to perform their functions properly

Macro-minerals include potassium, calcium, chloride and phosphorus. Sulfur, magnesium and sodium are other minerals that are needed in large quantities in the body.

9) **a:** Zinc, fluoride and iron

Trace minerals, unlike macro-minerals, are needed in large quantities. Examples of trace minerals are fluoride, zinc and iron. Other examples are selenium, manganese and cobalt. We can get these minerals by consuming a wide range of food that is rich in minerals.

10) **d:** All of the above

Water has many benefits. It helps prevent constipation and urinary tract infections. It also lubricates body organs, removes toxins and transports nutrients across the body.

11) **d:** To be in shape and stay healthy

Weight control is beneficial to individuals who are struggling with weight gain. It helps them stay healthy.

12) **a:** Soluble fiber and protein

Whole grains are rich in soluble fiber and protein. These are essential elements that support weight loss.

13) **c:** Because they have low energy density

Although all fruits are sugary, they are not as harmful as man-made sugars. Unlike man-made sugars, fruits have low energy density that makes them a lot healthier than synthetic sugars.

14) **a:** Nutrients, protein and fiber

Hypertensive patients should stay away from any type of food with the potential to increase their blood pressure.

15) **a:** A lack of sufficient lactase to break down and digest lactose

Someone who is lactase intolerant does not have enough lactase to break down and digest lactose consumed through foods and beverages. Such individuals may develop symptoms such as vomiting, bloating, stomach cramps and diarrhea.

16) **c:** They contain the right amount of enzymes to neutralize the effect of lactose

Lactose-free products are healthy for lactose-sensitive people because such products contain the right amount of enzymes the body needs to neutralize the effects of lactose.

17) **d:** Medical conditions that can affect the patient emotionally and health-wise

Eating disorders impact people's eating behaviors and adversely affect their emotions, health and ability to function properly. Eating disorders are considered a mental health condition that can be treated only by psychological and medical experts.

18) **d:** Unusual obsession with one's weight

Eating disorders are usually triggered by an unusual obsession with one's weight, food or body shape. The obsession can cause patients to develop some unhealthy eating habits that may have a lasting negative effect on their health and personality if not appropriately treated.

19) **c:** An eating disorder common to people who always consider themselves overweight

People with the medical condition always view themselves as overweight, although that may be far from the truth. In some cases, anorexia nervosa patients are actually underweight.

20) **b:** An eating disorder common to people irrespective of their age

Rumination disorder is a disorder that is common to people of all ages. This voluntary eating disorder can develop at any stage of the victim's life: infancy, childhood or adulthood. While infants get over this condition naturally, adults and children require professional assistance to resolve the problem.

21) **c:** Look for an appropriate and visible vein

Look for the appropriate and clearly visible vein before you apply the tourniquet. Apply the tourniquet about three to four inches above the site you wish to use for the venipuncture.

22) **b:** 70% alcohol swab
Although there may be an array of alcohol swabs and other disinfectants to choose from, the best disinfectant for a venipuncture site is 70% alcohol swab. Disinfecting the site is easy with this product.

23) **d:** A dermal puncture requires less precision than a venipuncture

A major difference between a dermal puncture and a venipuncture for taking blood samples is that a dermal puncture requires less precision than a venipuncture. Thus, health workers prefer dermal punctures to venipunctures when taking blood samples from infants.

24) **a:** It takes a longer processing time than a venipuncture

While dermal puncture is a popular blood sample technique, it takes a longer processing time than a venipuncture.

25) **a:** The collection technique and timing

The collection technique and timing are two important factors that determine the type of information that can be derived from urine tests. Different collection techniques yield different results. Also important is the time of the day the sample is taken.

26) **b:** First morning specimen

The first morning specimen is the specimen-taking technique that guarantees concentrated urine. This urine specimen is taken in the morning. The collected urine sample is usually more concentrated, thanks to the long duration of urine in the bladder overnight.

27) **b:** 8-hour specimen

The first morning specimen technique is otherwise known as an 8-hour specimen. This is named after how long the patient sleeps before the urine sample is taken. Remember, some experts recommend a minimum of eight hours of sleep every night.

28) **a:** Specimens should be transported in glass containers

Specimen collection is regulated by some guidelines. For instance, collection tubes must be properly labeled for easy identification. A transporting container should be used once and discarded. The containers should be clean and free of particles. Glass containers are not ideal for transporting specimens.

29) **c:** By their chemical activity and conditions treated by the drug

Drugs are grouped into different classes. The classification parameters are the conditions the drug is designed to treat and its chemical activity. Each class has distinct effects, characteristics and side effects.

30) **b:** Depressants that affect the central nervous system

Barbiturates are central nervous system depressants whose major symptoms, when taken reasonably, are a huge sense of relaxation and euphoria. Barbiturates are also known as downers. They are addictive substances that are sometimes abused.

31) **d:** Drugs that can increase a patient's alertness temporarily

Stimulants are drugs that people take to increase their alertness temporarily. They are available as tablets or capsules and are used in different ways. Some users snort them, while some inject them in liquid form or simply crush them and consume them.

32) **a:** Increased alertness and the desire to talk excessively

Stimulants have many side effects. The desire to talk excessively and increased alertness are two of them. Other side effects include increased heart rate, reduced appetite and euphoria.

33) **d:** All of the above

Another class of inhalants used for psychoactive effects on consumers is nitrites. Room deodorizers, video head cleaners and leather cleaners are examples of inhaled nitrites.

34) **c:** Both A and B

Some commercial household gases are used as inhalants. Notable examples include propane tanks, whipped cream aerosol and butane lighters. Some anesthesia gases such as ether and chloroform are used for the same purpose.

35) **a:** Delayed behavioral development and liver damage

Inhalants have both short-term and long-term side effects. Some of their long-term side effects are liver damage and delayed behavioral development. Kidney damage and brain damage resulting from insufficient oxygen flow to the brain are two other long-term effects.

36) **a:** Their ability to change a user's thoughts and emotions

Hallucinogens are used for both recreational purposes and religious rituals. Users take advantage of hallucinogens' ability to change their emotions and thoughts.

37) **a:** Marijuana

Marijuana is the most popular illegal drug used around the world. This mood-altering drug is classified as a Schedule 1 controlled substance due to its huge impact on nearly every body organ.

38) **b:** Over 120 compounds with distinct properties

Cannabis is made up of over 120 compounds with distinct properties derived from different parts of the cannabis sativa plant. The drug can be used for a wide range of purposes and can affect users adversely.

39) **a:** Sleep disturbances, chronic pain and muscle spasticity

Medical marijuana can be used to treat an array of ailments that include chronic pain, sleep disturbances and muscle spasticity. This form of the drug is not considered illegal in the United States.

40) **c:** Pain relievers that work on the nervous system
Opioids are a class of drugs that relieve pain by acting on the nervous system. The opium poppy plant is the primary source of opioids, and the drug can have a variety of effects on the user.

41) **b:** Between 8°C and 15°C

Medications are stored under different conditions. The appropriate storage temperature for medications that need to be kept cool is between 8°C and 15°C. That temperature range will sustain the drugs' potency.

42) **b:** An exaggeration of the therapeutic effect of a drug

This refers to the exaggeration of the therapeutic effect of the administered drug on the user. It occurs when the drug seemingly overperforms, leading to some side effects.

43) **c:** An adverse drug reaction that is triggered by some mechanisms that are not yet understood

An idiosyncratic adverse drug reaction refers to an adverse drug reaction that is triggered by some mechanisms that are not yet understood. Until they are better understood, idiosyncratic adverse drug reactions are unpredictable.

44) **c:** People whose parents are allergic to some drugs may react adversely

Hereditary factors may also play a huge role in some people's response to drugs. If your family has a history of allergies to certain drugs, you are more likely to respond negatively to such drugs too, increasing your adverse reactions to them.

45) **b:** Certain diseases and ailments

Adverse drug reactions can be triggered by several factors. Ailments and certain diseases are two such factors. Other factors that can trigger such reactions are hereditary factors, age and drug factors.

46) **d:** Section 6

If you need diagnostic product information, this is the right *Physicians' Desk Reference* section for that. The information includes the manufacturer's name, arranged alphabetically. The diagnostic guidelines for each drug that is not accompanied by official package information are available in this section.

47) **d:** Section 2

This *Physicians' Desk Reference* section contains page numbers for drugs. Generic name and brand name are used for the pagination. You will find this section useful when looking for unfamiliar drug names.

48) **c:** Vaginal route and nasal route

Drugs are administered in different ways. Some commonly used routes are oral administration, subcutaneous route, intramuscular route and vaginal route. The administration route is determined by the type of drug and its intended purpose.

49) **b:** Sprains and abrasions

Sprains and abrasions are some minor injuries that may require first aid.

50) **c:** When a foreign object lodges in someone's throat

An adult or a young child can experience choking when a foreign object lodges in the windpipe or throat and blocks airflow. This is usually caused by food in adults, while young children may fall victim after swallowing a foreign object.

51) **d:** All of the above

Some common choking signs include talking difficulties, breathing difficulties, flushed skin, lips turning blue, loss of consciousness and skin turning blue. As the throat is blocked, airflow to the victim's brain is stopped, leading to the medical conditions listed above.

52) **b:** Stand behind the person and bend him/her at the waist

One of the ways you can help someone who is choking on something is by standing behind the person and bending him/her at the waist. Then proceed with other first aid techniques as outlined earlier in this book.

53) **c:** Apply pressure to the affected area with a clean cloth

When treating a bleeding patient, the first step you can take to stop the bleeding is to apply pressure to the affected area with a clean cloth. Then you can proceed to the other steps as outlined in this book.

54) **c:** To reduce the flow of blood

Raising the affected area above the heart is an important step to take when treating a bleeding patient. Raising the area will reduce blood flow. Then implement other strategies that will stop the bleeding completely.

55) **a:** If the patient feels feverish or may be bleeding internally

Seek help if the patient may be bleeding internally or feels feverish. The input of a qualified doctor may be the difference between life and death for the patient.

56) **b:** A sudden decrease in someone's body temperature

Intense cold can have a damaging effect on people's health. It can lead to a huge drop in the patient's overall temperature, a condition medically known as hypothermia.

57) **b:** Wrapping the affected area with a soft and loose cloth

Frostbite occurs when someone's cells are frozen as a result of prolonged exposure to cold. To treat a frostbite victim, wrap the affected area with a soft and loose cloth. Call for assistance without delay.

58) **d:** None of the above

When treating a hypothermia patient, do not warm the person's arms and legs. Do not offer cigarettes or alcohol. While heating the person with a heating lamp or a hot bath may seem logical, it is not advisable.

59) **c:** An injury or death caused by swallowing harmful gases or drugs

Poisoning is death or injury caused by inhaling, swallowing or touching chemicals, some harmful drugs, gases or venom. Injecting harmful chemicals can also lead to poisoning.

60) **b:** The type of poison consumed

Treating a poison victim without knowing the type of poison the person has consumed or has been exposed to is not advisable. To determine the most effective antidote to give a poison victim, you need to know the type of poison. You cannot treat lead poisoning the same way you would treat food poisoning, for instance.

61) **c:** Flush the eye with lukewarm water

When someone is poisoned in the eye, flush the affected eye with lukewarm water gently for about 15 minutes. The water will flush the poison out of the affected eye.

62) **a:** Pill bottles, the packages or the pill container

When you call an ambulance for a patient who has been poisoned, the pill container or package may be necessary to help the medical team make the right treatment decision.

63) **b:** An option that should not be considered due to its high risk

Inducing vomiting with syrup of ipecac in patients who have been poisoned is not considered a medically appropriate response. While this practice was endorsed some years back, experts have now determined it causes more harm than good.

64) **b:** It enables you to understand the patient's medication

An asthmatic may have a treatment regimen. If you ask for such a plan, you will be better prepared to assist the victim.

65) **b:** Remove an embedded stinger by scraping the surface gently

Remove an embedded stinger and other things like ticks by scraping the surface gently with a flat-edged object. Do not use tweezers for the removal, as that tends to release more venom as you squeeze the area affected by the sting.

66) **d:** All of the above

Insect stings or bites can be treated by medications such as crotamiton lotion, antihistamine tablets, ibuprofen, paracetamol and hydrocortisone ointment.

67) **c:** Both A and B

Acetaminophen and ibuprofen are both useful for treating headaches, but acetaminophen is a bit more effective.

68) **d:** Restraining the person's movements

When someone suffers from seizures, you can assist them in regaining consciousness and reducing accidental injury by loosening anything that may impede breathing. You should not insert any object in a seizure victim's mouth. Do not restrain the victim in any way. However, you should remove nearby objects that may cause injury.

69) **b:** A medical condition that refers to loss of heart function, breathing and consciousness

Cardiac arrest is a sudden loss of breathing, heart function and consciousness. This medical condition is usually triggered when the heart experiences a sudden electrical disturbance.

70) **b:** Heart attack is a halting of blood flow to the heart muscle, while cardiac arrest is a loss of breathing and consciousness

Cardiac arrests and heart attacks are often erroneously used interchangeably. However, they are different medical conditions. A heart attack is a medical condition that is characterized by the halting of blood flow to the heart muscle, while cardiac arrest refers to the loss of breathing and consciousness.

71) **c:** Compression

When treating sprains, the affected area must be compressed for two consecutive days. Do this with an elastic compression bandage.

72) **d:** Waiting for a physician to perform CPR

When you are faced with emergencies, provide first aid while awaiting the arrival of a physician. If the patient shows no signs of life, perform CPR immediately. The patient may die while waiting for the physician if you do not act swiftly.

73) **b:** Ligament injuries caused by torn ligament fibers

Torn ligament fibers are the cause of ligament injuries. Some common signs and symptoms of sprains are difficulty moving the affected area, swelling in the affected area and pain in the joint or muscle, among others.

74) **c:** The type of accident

The type of accident you are faced with determines your response. You cannot apply the same treatment to all forms of accidents.

75) **c:** Between 30 seconds and two minutes

Seizures usually last between 30 seconds and two minutes.

76) **c:** It may damage the heart and lungs

Massaging someone suffering from hypothermia will not solve the problem and will instead compound it. Massaging a cold body may damage the lungs and heart.

77) **d:** Waiting for permission for the patient or relatives before rendering assistance

When offering first aid during emergencies, do not wait for permission from the patient or relatives before providing the necessary assistance. However, you can check the scene for signs of potential danger and call for medical assistance if necessary.

78) **a:** To prevent a health condition from deteriorating

Emergency situations may put people's lives or health at risk. Offering first aid will prevent a patient's condition from deteriorating.

79) **a:** The drug's formula and how it works

Drugs are administered in a variety of ways. The best administration method is determined by the drug's formula, as stipulated by the manufacturer.

80) **c:** Estrogen

A typical example of a vaginally administered drug is estrogen. Menopausal women use this drug to treat vaginal medical conditions, such as soreness, dryness and redness. It is administered vaginally.

81) **a:** Upper arm and thigh

The target destination for injecting the drug is the muscles of the thigh, the upper arm or the buttocks.

82) **a:** Oral administration

Oral drug administration is a common administration route for drugs that can be used as capsules, liquids, chewable tablets or tablets. It can be argued that the oral route is the safest, most convenient and least expensive drug administration method.

83) **b:** Section 2

This section of the *Physicians' Desk Reference* contains page numbers for drugs. Generic names and brand names are used for the pagination. You will find this section useful when looking for unfamiliar drug names.

84) **b:** The Food and Drug Administration and pharmaceutical companies

The *Physicians' Desk Reference* is an annually published reference guide for physicians. The book is a list of all the licensed drugs in the United States. These drugs are approved by the Food and Drug Administration, and information about them is published with the assistance of the pharmaceutical companies in the country.

85) **a:** Age and hereditary factors

People react adversely to drugs for several reasons. Some factors that are responsible for such negative reactions include age and heredity. Young people, infants and the elderly are more prone to such reactions than middle-aged people. The same goes for people with a family history of allergies to some drugs.

86) **d:** All of the above

Some factors that may affect a drug's potency are heat, light and moisture.

87) **b:** They block pain signals between the brain and the body

Opioids are used for treating moderate pain due to their ability to block pain signals between the brain and the body.

88) **d:** None of the above

Hallucinogens are available as PCP, ayahuasca, mescaline, psilocybin, D-lysergic acid diethylamide and dimethyltryptamine.

89) **c:** Hallucinogens

Hallucinogens have been used for years for spiritual and healing purposes thanks to their ability to change a user's thoughts, emotions and consciousness.

90) **a:** Insomnia and seizures

Some common ailments that can be treated with depressants are insomnia and seizures. Depressants are also used to treat depression, social phobias and obsessive-compulsive disorder.

91) **d:** Psychoactive drugs for treating insomnia and anxiety

Benzodiazepines are a class of psychoactive drugs used for treating insomnia and anxiety. As a result, they are ranked among the most widely used depressants in the United States.

92) **a:** Central nervous system depressants

Barbiturates are central nervous system depressants that give users a sense of euphoria and relaxation. They affect a user's sleep patterns and suppress REM sleep. Barbiturates are addictive.

93) **b:** Read and follow storage instructions

When reagents are not properly stored, they may not work as expected, and that can have a huge impact on the result.

94) **c:** Accuracy and reliability of the result of the analysis

The usefulness of an analysis is dependent on the accuracy and reliability of the result. If the result is flawed, such a result is of no use in helping determine a treatment for a patient.

95) **a:** Through the addition of preservatives or refrigeration

When the urine has been collected over a 24-hour period, it can be preserved with the addition of the right preservative. In the absence of a preservative, the collected urine can be refrigerated for as long as necessary.

96) **c:** It provides false and misleading information

While the random specimen technique is popular among health workers, its major shortcoming is that it can provide false and misleading information, especially if the specimen is overdiluted.

97) **c:** It may result in hemolysis or blood clotting

A dermal puncture is more time-consuming than a venipuncture. This may have a huge impact on the outcome of whatever test is done with the collected specimen. For instance, the delay may result in hemolysis or blood clotting.

98) **d:** Drinking water and freshly squeezed juices

People can stay hydrated by drinking plenty of liquids throughout the day. Aside from increasing their water consumption, they should also hydrate with freshly squeezed juice. This will increase their body's vitamin level as well as prevent other health problems that may arise from dehydration.

99) **d:** Water

Water is one of the most important nutrients needed by the body. Dehydration may cause impaired physical functioning and headaches, as well as hamper a person's mental abilities.

100) **d:** It leads to frequent urination

Water serves different functions in the body. It lubricates body organs, serves as a shock absorber and removes toxins. Water also prevents constipation, transports nutrients and prevents dehydration.

Conclusion

Taking the CMA Exam is the first step towards achieving your career goals as a medical assistant. Therefore, preparing for the test is extremely important.

This guide contains everything you need to prepare for the exam.

Remembers the procedure for registering for the exam and the rules of the testing center, including what ID to take with you.

Familiarize yourself with the first aid procedures for different emergencies. Know common medical terminologies, suffixes and prefixes.

Understand the requirements for appointment scheduling.

The practice sections are designed as a review for the test. Take them seriously. Go over them as many times as necessary to feel comfortable with the information.

Made in the USA
Las Vegas, NV
10 March 2021